everyday eating for babies & children

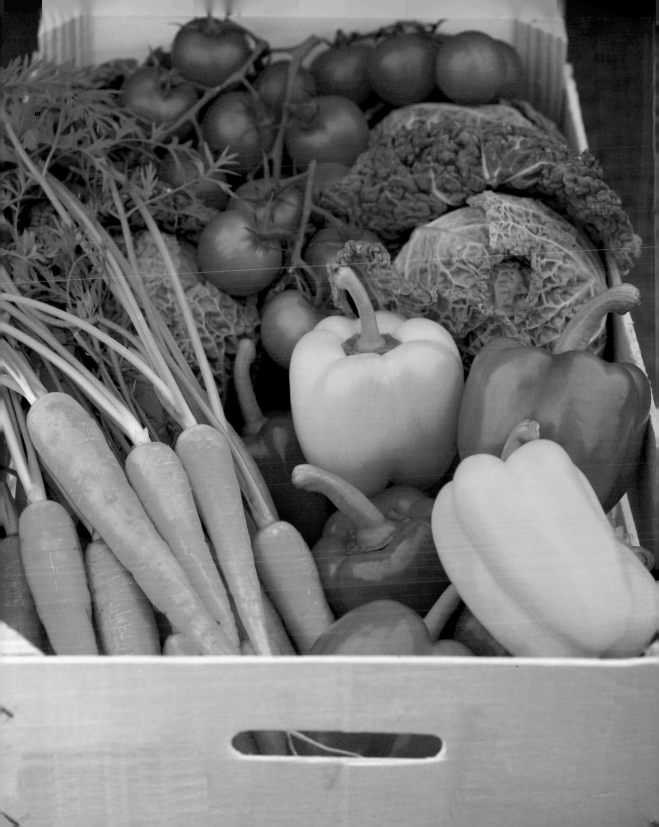

Judith Wills

everyday eating for babies & children

Collins

First published in 2006 by Collins
an imprint of HarperCollinsPublishers
77–85 Fulham Palace Road, London, W6 8JB

Material in this book was previously published
in *Children's Food Bible* by Judith Wills.

Text © 2006 Judith Wills
Photography and design © 2006 HarperCollinsPublishers

Editor: Janet Illsley
Design: Smith & Gilmour, London
Photographer: Nikki English

A CIP catalogue record for this book is available from the
British Library.

ISBN 0-00-721527-4

Colour reproduction by Colourscan, Singapore
Printed by Printing Express Ltd, Hong Kong

Notes

The symbols alongside the recipes indicate
which age group they are suitable for:

6 mths+ Suitable for infants and children
over 6 months

12 mths+ Suitable for children over 1 year

5 years+ Suitable for children over 5 years

Each recipe has a guide to suitability for
special diets, to help you choose meals for
children with particular needs: vegetarian;
vegan; nut- and seed-free; wheat- and
gluten-free; dairy-free.

Nutritional information next to each recipe
highlights those nutrients the dish is a good
source of.

The number of servings alongside each recipe
relates to the youngest group the recipe is
suitable for. If making the recipe for older
children it will serve fewer than stated, so you
will need to adjust the quantities accordingly.
In any case, the required portion size will
depend on your child's appetite and activity
level. Regard the number of servings as
an approximate guide only.

Contents

Introduction 6

From weaning to 12 months 8
Successful weaning 10
Choosing the right foods for your baby 16
Drinks for infants 24
Eating plans 26
Recipes 32

The toddler & pre-school child's diet 48
Nutritional needs of toddlers and pre-school children 50
The food pyramid 52
Feeding problems 55
Eating plans 58
Recipes 68

Starting school: new influences on diet 104
Nutritional needs of young primary school children 106
The school day 110
Encouraging healthy eating 114
Weight issues 117
Eating plans 119
Recipes 122

A–Z of child health & diet 132
Essential information on nutrition and food safety;
disorders and possible diet solutions

Index 220
Contacts 224

Introduction

What is it that every parent wants the most for his or her child? I believe it is good health. We want our children to be healthy now, to stay healthy throughout childhood, and to grow into healthy adults with a long life ahead. And one of the most significant – and simple – ways to achieve this is through diet. What you choose to feed your children and, later, what advice you give them about making their own choices will have wide-ranging effects on their physical and even mental health throughout life.

In theory, feeding our children well shouldn't be a problem since the volume of research into, and information about, children's diet and health has never been greater. But ironically, statistics show that a high proportion of children's diets in the West are having negative, rather than positive, effects on their health and the situation is getting worse.

According to the Royal College of Paediatrics, we are raising a generation of children who are overweight but poorly nourished. Children are eating too much saturated fat, far too much sugar and salt, and only 50% of the optimum amount of fruits and vegetables. Some children don't eat any citrus fruit at all, only about half have salad and only around a third eat any leafy greens. Oily fish, whole grains and natural yoghurt hardly figure at all in our children's diets. On the other hand, their consumption of sweets, crisps, fizzy drinks and takeaway fast foods has increased dramatically. No wonder that four out of five parents worry about their children's diet, but feel guilty because they don't invest enough time or effort in improving it.

One government health minister anticipates that the current young generation may not live as long as their parents – a prediction endorsed by various child health and obesity specialists. But why have our eating habits changed for the worst? Experts cite the modern fast food culture, peer pressure and advertising, in addition to the poor monitoring and standard of school meals, and the decline of parental influence and home-cooked family meals.

As a direct consequence of poor diet and a decline in physical activity among children, we are now experiencing record levels of childhood obesity. In this country, the number of overweight children has doubled in a decade to nearly 20%.

In turn, poor diet and overweight have led to a rapidly increasing incidence of 'modern' illnesses such as diabetes and heart disease in young adults, while early signs of artery disease are showing in children as young as 7 years of age. It is also becoming apparent that many other childhood complaints, such as asthma, behavioural problems and eczema may be influenced by diet.

But even the most health-conscious parents often feel that they are battling against the tactics of the huge multinational food conglomerates, who are more concerned with healthy accounts than healthy eating. Indeed these companies often seem to have a diametrically opposed view to that of the nutrition experts about what children should eat. There isn't so much profit in fruit and vegetables!

But it is becoming clear that we *do* have a choice. There is increasing publicity about the need for good, healthy food for our children. Slowly, very slowly, government is getting the message and as a consequence we should see improvement in how schools sell food and teach healthy eating, and in legislation for better control of food labelling, safety, marketing and so on.

Meanwhile, this book is my own contribution. My aim has been to produce an unbiased reference resource for parents, hopefully answering all the 'whats', 'whys' and 'how-to's' that you regularly find yourself asking. This first part of the book provides advice for parents at each stage of a young child's development and is divided into three sections – from weaning to 12 months, the toddler and pre-school years, then the early years at primary school.

These chapters highlight the changing dietary needs of children as they grow and as their circumstances alter, and address the different eating problems that are typical for each age group and how they may affect health. From allergies in toddlers to healthy eating at school, you will find help in this section. There is also plenty of advice on meal planning, with 'blueprint' eating plans for each age group, including specific advice for feeding the vegetarian child.

The information in these chapters is best used in conjunction with the A–Z of child health & diet, which forms the second part of the book. This provides more detailed advice on dozens of topics – cross-references on most pages will lead you to the relevant areas of the A–Z. You will also find a list of websites and contact details for food, diet and health organisations at the back of the book.

Most of us are fortunate enough to have easy access to the food needed for a varied, balanced, interesting and healthy diet. Broaden your knowledge about food and related health issues and you will have the confidence – and the power – to give your children a healthy and enjoyable diet, right through their growing years.

Judith Wills

From weaning to 12 months

When our children are small, we have a never-to-be-repeated chance to instill good eating habits into them – as well as the opportunity to encourage them to enjoy food and feel good about their relationship with it. Good nutrition is key t o the future health and development of any child. It is probable that every child's short- and long-term health can be improved if parents wean at the right time, and then provide a nutritious and suitable diet from weaning onwards.

While it isn't necessary to be overprotective about what your children eat as babies and infants, almost all the research shows that this is the ideal time to encourage them to develop healthy tastes in food – and to do so is probably easier than you might imagine. The first few years are, in effect, the only time that you will have the opportunity for 100% control over what your children eat and drink. Getting your infant off to a good start is what this chapter is all about.

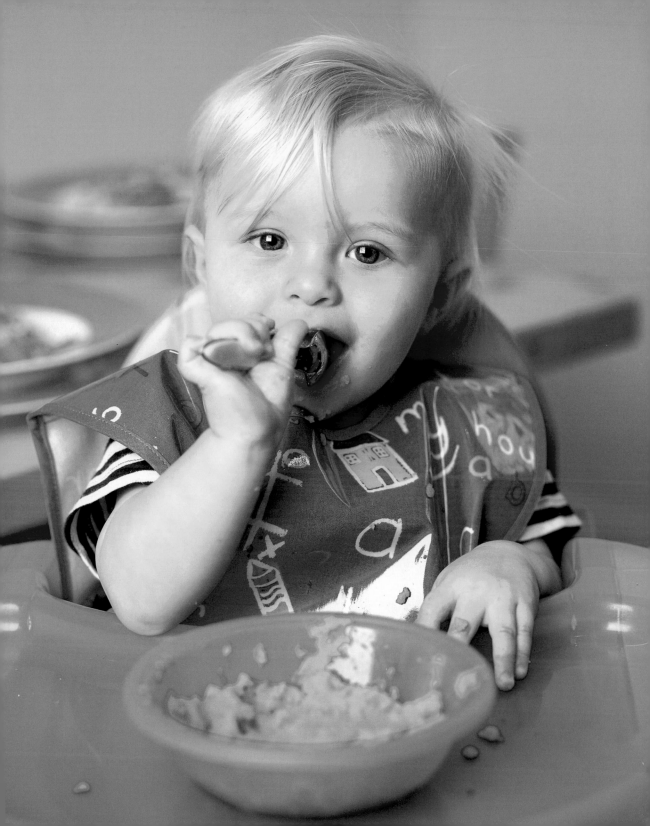

Successful weaning

A baby's first natural food is breast milk. In the UK, according to the Department of Health, 71% of new mothers breast-feed their babies for at least 2 weeks. Bottle feeding with a formula based on cows' or soya milk is an alternative. If possible, however, you should try to breast-feed, as there are many natural advantages to be had.

Studies have shown that, in addition to building up the immune system, there is evidence that breast milk can also help visual development and improve mental skills and brain power (though formula milk with added essential fats has been shown to produce similar results). The long-chain fatty acids in breast milk could also protect your baby against high blood pressure, helping to prevent heart disease and strokes in later life.

Advantages of breast milk
- Hygienic, temperature-controlled – and free!
- Protects your baby against infection
- Helps build a healthy immune system
- May aid visual development and mental skills
- Protects against high blood pressure
- May protect against becoming overweight

The current consensus of expert opinion is that breast or bottle milk should be the only food you provide for your infant for at least the first 4 months, and that weaning before this age is detrimental. Indeed, the UK Department of Health advises women that breast-feeding as the sole source of nutrition is preferable for the first 6 months. The British Nutrition Foundation (BNF) suggests that it may be time for weaning when the baby's weight reaches 7kg (or doubles from birth weight).

Recommendations on feeding infants
(Uk Department of Health)
- Breast milk is the best form of nutrition for infants
- Exclusive breast-feeding is recommended for the first 6 months of an infant's life
- The recommended age for the introduction of solid foods for infants is 6 months
- Breast-feeding (and/or breast milk substitutes, if used) should continue beyond the first 6 months, along with appropriate types and amounts of solid foods

All infants should be managed individually so that insufficient growth or other outcomes are not ignored.

Early weaning problems
There are good reasons for not weaning early:

Baby's digestion The digestive system and kidneys of young babies may not be able to cope readily with solid foods.

Development of allergies Later weaning may help to prevent infant and childhood allergies from developing.

Tendency towards obesity There is some evidence to show that children weaned on to solids at an early age tend to be fatter.

Late weaning problems

Although early weaning is not advisable, neither is late weaning if delayed much beyond 6 months, as it has been linked with:

Malnutrition Breast milk alone is unlikely to provide all the nutrients and calories that a growing baby needs after 6 months. There is little iron or vitamin D in breast milk, for example, and by 6 months the baby's own stores will be used up. (With formula milk, this isn't a problem.)

Slow development of eating skills Babies may find it harder to develop the correct chewing response or learn to accept 'lumpy' food if weaning doesn't start at around 6 months.

Development of fussy eating Experts claim that children exposed to a wide variety of tastes and textures between 6 and 9 months are less likely to become faddy eaters.

See also: Allergies and infants p22, Feeding problems p55, Food allergies p162, Fussy eating and food refusal p174.

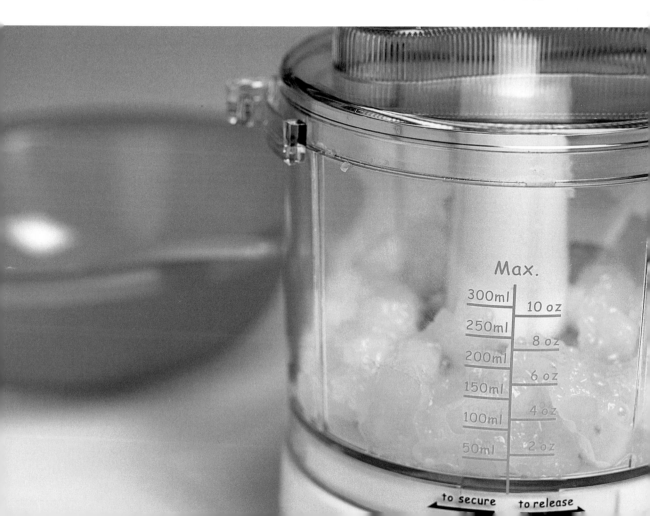

Foods to wean your infant on

A child is described as an infant from birth to aged 12 months. During this time your baby is growing rapidly and so he or she will need enough calories from fats, carbohydrates and protein, and a range of vitamins and minerals. As long as you give your baby a range of suitable foods from each of the food groups (see opposite) and he or she appears to be thriving and growing well, you are almost certainly providing them with a nutritionally balanced diet.

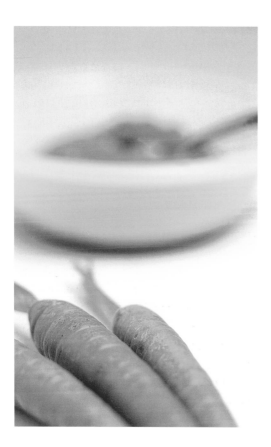

In general, your infant's fat intake (as a proportion of his or her total calorie intake) should be higher than that for an adult. Breast and formula milks are about 50% fat.

The first weaning food is most often baby rice mixed to a creamy consistency with a little breast or formula milk, or boiled water, and served slightly warm. Vegetable purées can be introduced after a week or two – the sweeter vegetables, such as carrot, sweet potato and squash, are usually very well received. Fruit purées, such as apple, pear and banana, can then follow. All purées should be lump-free at this stage, to avoid choking or refusal, and they should be introduced one at a time in small amounts on the end of a flat plastic baby spoon. You'll find further advice about making purées on page 14.

Once your baby has been taking solids for several weeks you can introduce other foods to provide a more varied diet. By around 7 months, most babies will enjoy a range of cereals, mild fish, eggs, dairy produce, chicken, turkey and a variety of fruit and veg – purées can be slightly thicker.

By the time they are 9–12 months old, most babies will accept food that is more textured and will enjoy eating finger foods, such as cooked carrot or broccoli sticks or pieces of ripe banana.

After he or she reaches the age of 1, your baby will begin to enjoy meals similar to those that the rest of the family are eating.

Feeding infants after weaning

After weaning, your child regularly needs a variety of foods from each of the following four food groups:

Milk and dairy foods These provide calcium for bone growth and health, protein for muscle growth, fat, carbohydrate, vitamins and a variety of minerals.

Meat, fish, eggs, pulses These provide protein, fat and a wide range of vitamins and minerals. Pulses also contain carbohydrate and fibre.

Cereals, bread and potatoes The starch foods provide an important source of energy (calories) in the diet as well as fibre, vitamins and minerals.

Fruit and vegetables These provide your child's main source of vitamin C and other vitamins and minerals, and also contain important plant chemicals (phytochemicals) and fibre.

See also: Phytochemicals p195.

Good sources of iron for the newly weaned infant

- Lean red meat
- Pulses (lentils, chickpeas, etc.)
- Eggs
- Dried apricots, prunes and other dried fruits
- Dark green vegetables, e.g. broccoli, spring greens

So long as an infant has a good quality, varied and balanced diet, vitamin and mineral supplements should not be necessary.

The vegetarian infant

The parents of infants who are vegetarian may have to work a little harder to ensure they don't fall short on iron, as meat is the main dietary source of easily absorbed iron for non-vegetarians. Lentils and other pulses, dried fruits, eggs and leafy greens are all good sources. Iron absorption is helped if the iron-rich food is eaten with a vitamin C-rich food or drink. High-fibre foods can hinder absorption. Dairy produce should provide sufficient protein and calcium in the diet and a wide variety of cereals, pulses, fruits and veg should provide all the vitamins and minerals.

If your infant is vegan (eating no dairy produce or eggs either), you need to ensure that he or she receives enough calcium. Continue breast-feeding for as long as possible. Other good vegan sources of calcium are mineral-enriched soya formula, tofu, fortified baby breakfast cereals, leafy green vegetables and dried fruits. He or she may also need a vitamin B12 supplement unless you are feeding B12-fortified soya products or breakfast cereals.

Both vegetarian and vegan babies may benefit from a supplement of omega-3 (long-chain) fatty acids. These essential fats are vital for maintaining health and development, and our main source in the diet is usually oily fish, although breast milk contains variable amounts of essential fats and some formula feeds also contain added omega-3s. The main non-fish source is flaxseed (linseed) oil.

See also: Essential Fatty Acids p156, Supplements p208.

General tips on feeding infants

Meal routines Aim to get your infant settled into a three-meals-a-day routine, with breast or formula milk snacks in-between meals. Most infants exercise their own portion control, refusing food when they have had enough to eat.

Home-cooking or jars? Try to provide your infant with as many home-cooked meals as possible, as this is the best way for him or her to get accustomed to the flavours of family meals. However, commercial baby foods can be convenient from time to time, especially when travelling. Don't feel guilty for having a few jars as standbys!

Making purées It is easy to make your own purées, especially if you have an electric blender. First peel, chop and deseed the vegetable or fruit if necessary. If it requires cooking, steam or boil in a little unsalted water until tender, then drain. Whiz in an electric blender with a little breast or formula milk or boiled water, until you have a smooth, creamy consistency. Or push through a sieve or mouli or mash with the liquid. After a few weeks, gradually make the purées less liquid and less smooth. In this way you can slowly introduce your baby to texture in food.

Batch cooking This can save time and effort – freeze small portions of purées in ice trays, then bag them and defrost as necessary. Reheat thoroughly in a saucepan or the microwave and then allow to cool to the required temperature.

Food safety When preparing, cooking and feeding, keep your hands and equipment scrupulously clean.

Weight issues Although many people warm to 'chubby' babies, and infants do naturally have a higher body-fat percentage than adults, it is important that your baby doesn't put on too much weight in their first year. If you think that your infant may be too fat, take him or her to the doctor, who will arrange for the baby to be weighed and assessed by a professional, who should be able to advise you. Similarly, you should seek professional advice if you think your baby is not gaining enough weight.

See also: Food Safety p167.

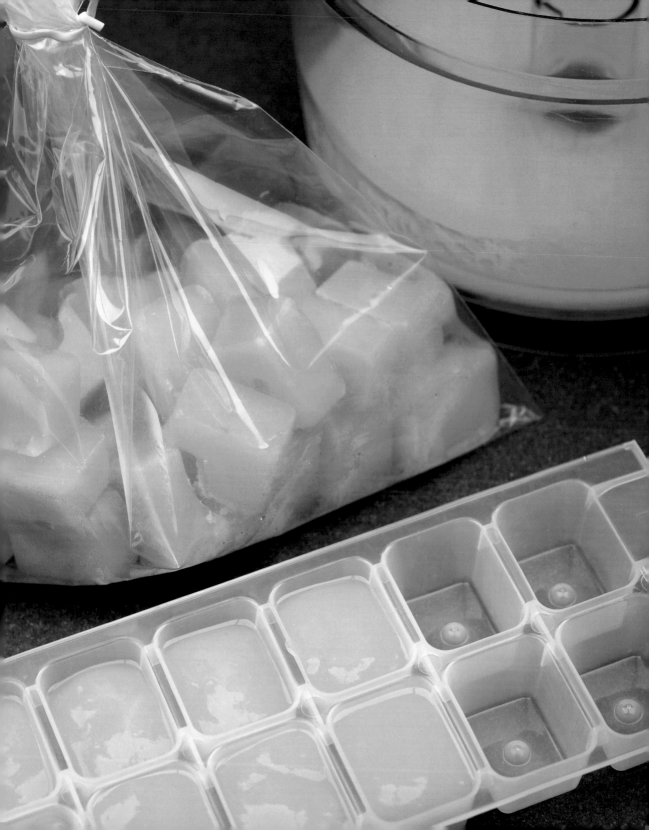

Choosing the right foods for your baby

It is important to follow official guidelines on which foods to offer and which to avoid giving your baby in infancy. Some foods can cause allergic reactions, others are difficult to digest, while others are unsuitable for small children for other reasons. The following guidelines should help you to decide what foods to offer and what foods to avoid at each stage from 6–12 months.

Suitable foods around 6 months

Suitable foods

At first, offer 1–2 small spoonfuls of baby rice halfway through a milk feed. Introduce mashed potato, polenta (fine cornmeal), puréed vegetables such as carrot and squash, puréed fruits such as apple and pear, and then purées of other fruits and vegetables, such as peas, parsnips, plums and bananas, as the early weeks of weaning progress. Small amounts of cooked meat, such as chicken, may be introduced to the purées towards the end of the first weaning period.

Foods to avoid

Don't ever add salt to baby foods, and only add sugar to sweeten sharp fruits.

Avoid all types of nuts but especially groundnuts (peanuts), seeds, grains containing gluten e.g. wheat, oats, barley and rye, eggs, cheese, yoghurt, cows' milk and other dairy foods, fish and shellfish, and citrus and berry fruits, as these are the most common allergens in infants.

Also avoid honey which can cause a type of food poisoning called infant botulism.

Don't give your baby offal or strong-tasting foods that he or she may not enjoy.

TIPS

Don't add baby rice or other foods to a drinks bottle as the baby may choke.

Introduce new foods one at a time, a little at a time. Your baby will dictate how much he or she wants to eat, usually just a couple of spoonfuls at this age.

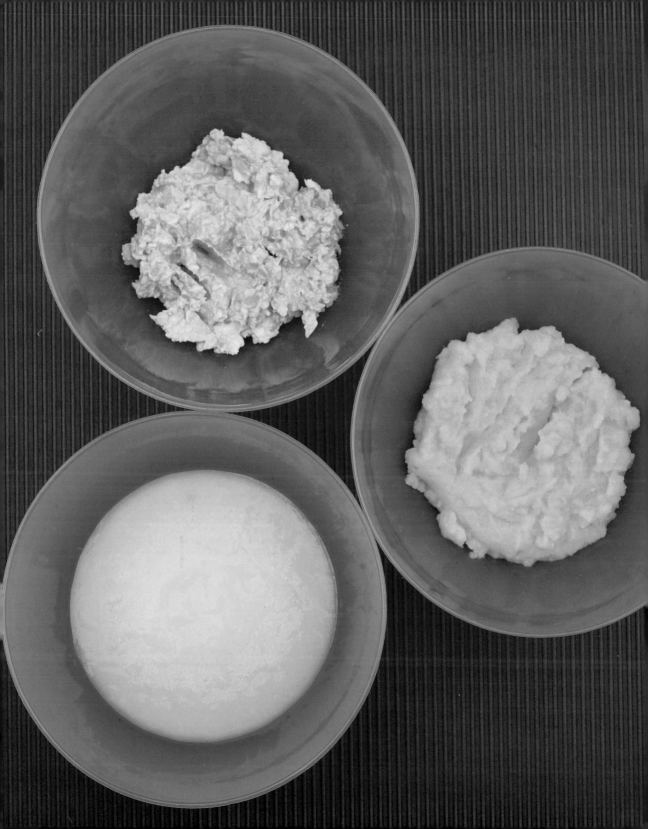

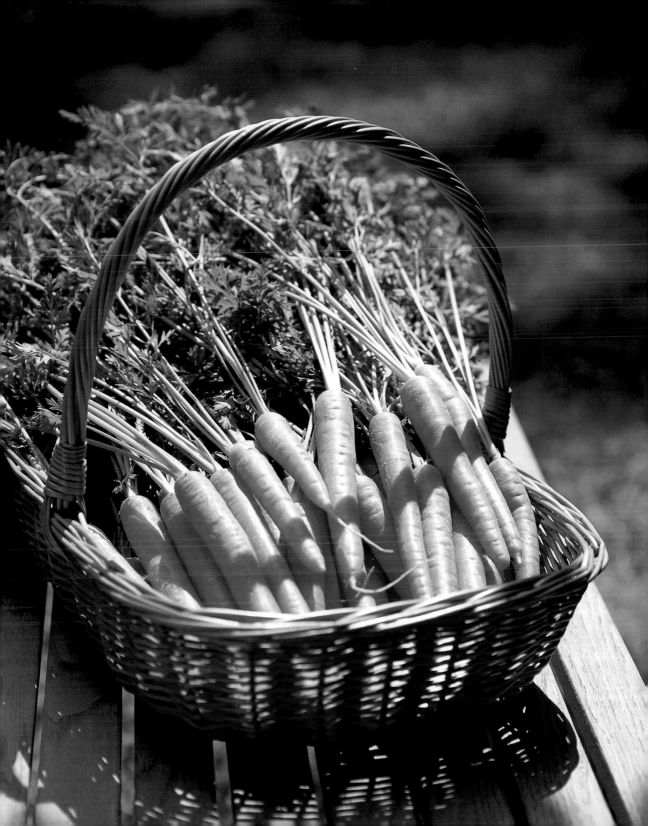

Suitable foods from 6–9 months

Suitable foods

This is the age to try many foods. Offer an increasing variety of fruits (e.g. avocado, papaya, melon, peach) and vegetables (e.g. cauliflower, swede, sweet potato, broccoli), along with some high-protein foods, such as red lentils and other dried pulses, chicken, turkey, white fish (like cod or coley), natural bio yoghurt, lean red meat. Gluten-containing grains – wheat, oats, barley and rye – are fine for most babies now, as are small amounts of hard cheese, such as Cheddar and pasteurized soft cheeses, hard-cooked egg yolk and small quantities of cows' milk as part of a dish (not as a drink). A tiny portion of offal can be given once a week – it is rich in iron, but contains high levels of vitamin A, too much of which can be dangerous for infants.

Foods to avoid

Groundnuts (peanuts) and other nuts, seeds, offal, egg white and uncooked or lightly cooked egg yolks, soft cheeses and blue cheeses, shark, swordfish or marlin, shellfish, added sugar except to sweeten sour fruits, added salt, honey.

TIPS

- Gradually make the purées a little thicker and with more texture, to encourage chewing.
- Between 7 and 9 months, gradually change from blended to mashed or well-minced food. Many babies are keen to eat their 'solid' meals at this age and slightly less interested in their milk.
- From 8 months, offer plenty of finger foods, such as slices of peeled fruits, lightly cooked broccoli or carrot, or fingers of bread or unsalted rice cakes or breadsticks. Some baby rusks contain added sugar and these are best avoided, so always read the label.

Suitable foods from 9–12 months

Suitable foods

Try reintroducing foods that your baby may not have enjoyed a few months ago – stronger tastes may be more acceptable now. All fruits and vegetables are suitable now – try sieved berry fruits, seedless satsumas, tomatoes. You can now offer egg white as well as yolk (well cooked), and it is a good time to try tiny amounts of oily fish such as tuna.

Foods to avoid

Groundnuts (peanuts) and other nuts, shark, swordfish or marlin, salty foods, foods containing much added sugar, sweets, soft and blue cheeses, shellfish, honey, raw or lightly cooked eggs.

TIPS

Always make sure that any fish is completely bone-free.

Your baby can eat with the family – mash or chop his or her food and don't add salt or use it in cooking.

Encourage the baby as much as possible to try to feed him- or herself.

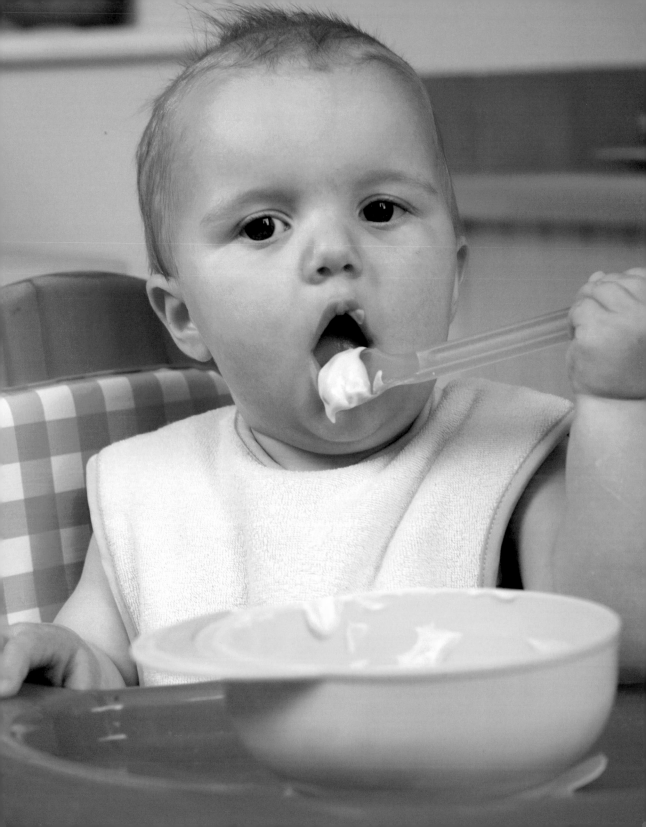

Allergies and infants

Several everyday foods that most infants can eat with no problem may cause an adverse reaction in some babies. Food intolerance (including allergy) is much more prevalent in babies and children up to the age of 5 than it is in other age groups – official estimates are that between 1 in 5 and 1 in 10 in this age group are affected by intolerance and 1–2% by 'true' allergy.

The foods most likely to cause an adverse reaction are cows' milk (up to 2% of infants are allergic to cows'-milk protein), egg (prevalence of actual allergy estimated in one recent study at 1.3%), soya, peanuts (groundnuts – but not groundnut oil) and other nuts, fish and shellfish. Wheat and other gluten-containing grains can cause coeliac disease in susceptible infants, while reports of allergy to sesame seeds are on the increase. Reactions have also been reported to citrus fruits, chicken, all dairy produce, goats' and ewes' milk, other seeds and exotic fruits, such as mango. Food additives may also cause allergic reactions.

The infants most susceptible to an allergic reaction or intolerance are those who have a family history (either parent or sibling) of allergy. Breast-feeding for up to 6 months will give some protection – and the mother may be advised to avoid the potentially allergenic foods while breast-feeding. For mothers who don't breast-feed and have infants who are allergic to cows' milk, various other infant formulas are available, such as soya formula (which can also cause allergy in approximately 5–10% of children who have a cows' milk allergy), or a hydrolysed milk formula. Unmodified goats' and sheep's milks are unsuitable for infants.

For susceptible infants, weaning on to solid foods before 6 months is strongly discouraged. None of the known common food allergens should be offered before 6 months at the earliest, according to the Department of Health, while other experts recommend avoidance of these foods for the first year.

Because not all adverse reactions to food occur in children with a family history of allergy, parents and carers of all infants are also advised to avoid foods that most commonly cause an adverse reaction until various age milestones are reached. Refer to the advice (on pages 16–20) for appropriate ages to introduce new foods.

Symptoms of a food allergy or intolerance can include vomiting, abdominal pain, diarrhoea, eczema, rashes, swelling (especially around the mouth), asthma and breathing difficulty.

A severe and immediate allergic reaction called anaphylaxis is a rare but possible occurrence – peanuts are the leading cause of anaphylactic shock and there is evidence that 'sensitisation' often occurs in the first year. About 1 in 200 children is thought to have a peanut allergy (though some experts put this figure much higher. In any case, peanuts and other nuts should never be fed to infants, as they can cause choking.

Most common allergenic foods

- Cows' milk
- Eggs
- Soya, peanuts (groundnuts) and other nuts
- Fish and shellfish

If you suspect that your infant does have a food allergy or intolerance, or you have any food allergy in your family and are thinking of becoming pregnant, are already pregnant or have an infant, you should go and get professional advice from your GP, who should, in turn, refer you to a State Registered Dietitian. The good news is that a high percentage of infants simply outgrow their food allergies, especially an allergy to cows' milk. Peanut allergy, however, is much less frequently outgrown and gluten intolerance is usually a lifelong disease.

Up to 90% of children will have outgrown an allergy to cows' milk by the age of 3, according to the Royal Society of Medicine.

Above all – don't panic! If you follow these guidelines, your baby has a 90%-plus chance of no adverse reactions to food at all. Don't go avoiding hundreds of different foods, other than those listed above, on the off-chance there might be a problem. Children need a wide variety of foods at this time and you could cause other problems, including fussy eating or even malnutrition. If you are ever at all worried about food allergies – see your doctor!

See also: Food Allergies p162.

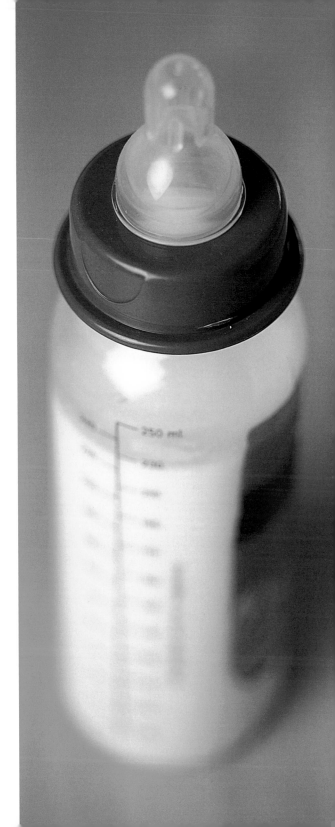

Drinks for infants

It is very important that infants have plenty of fluids. From weaning to 12 months the most suitable drink for your baby is still breast or formula milk. In the early days of weaning, a baby will still want milk at every meal and weaning foods will form a fairly small, but gradually increasing, part of his or her diet. It is best to start offering milk in a baby cup rather than a bottle as soon as you can when weaning begins. The baby can still have a bottle before bedtime up to one year old – if he or she needs it.

Aim to give your infant 600ml of breast or formula milk a day up to 1 year of age. 'Follow-on' formulas are available for babies over 6 months – for some babies these may be more suitable than early infant formula as they contain more nutrients – but if a wide variety of foods are being eaten, follow-on milk may not be necessary. Babies under one year old shouldn't be given ordinary cows', goats' or ewes' milk as a drink, as it doesn't contain enough nutrients.

If your baby seems to be thirsty, offer plain cooled boiled tap water. Avoid sparkling mineral water and any mineral waters with a high mineral content. For safety, bottled water still needs to be boiled until your baby is 6 months old.

If you want to give your infant any other drink, give him or her an occasional unsweetened fruit juice, well diluted with cooled boiled water, but in a cup rather than a bottle, as the sugars and acids in fruit juices can contribute to tooth decay. A high intake of fruit juice has also been linked with diarrhoea and overweight in infants. For children aged 1 year, it is recommended that the intake of fruit juice should be limited to no more than 170ml per day, so younger infants should be given rather less than this. Indeed, some paediatricians advise withholding all juice until at least 6 months of age.

- Avoid all drinks with added sugar or artificial sweeteners, and all caffeine-containing drinks which can hinder mineral absorption and may cause other problems.
- Don't leave your baby with a bottle of milk or juice – continual sucking of such drinks can cause tooth decay over time.
- Don't give infants juice at bedtime.

See also: Drinks p153, Milk p184, Teeth and Gums p209, Water p218.

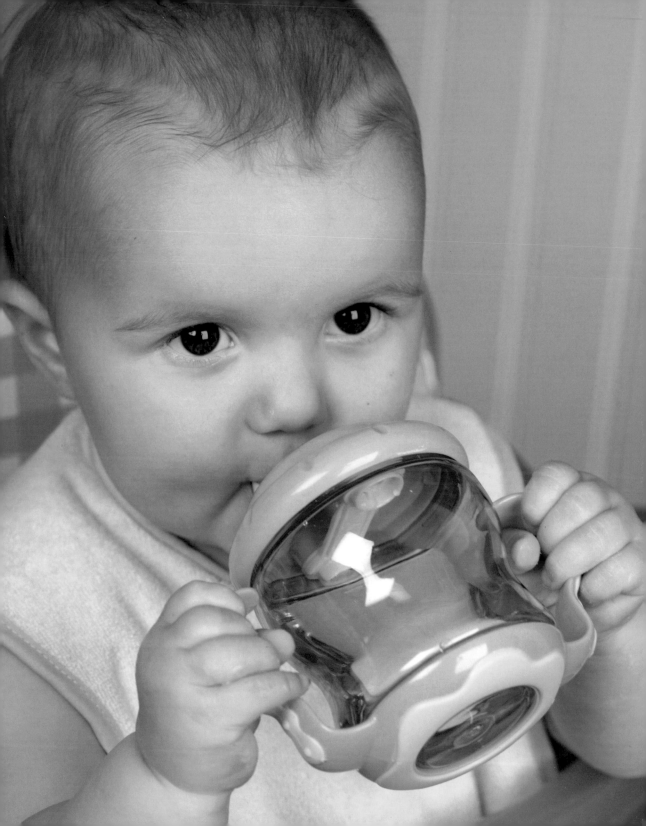

Planning your baby's meals

These eating plans are intended to help you plan your baby's meals at different stages of their development. They are flexible and intended as a guide rather than a rigid plan. The following guidelines apply:

- All milk feeds are breast or formula.
- All amounts are guidelines only; feed amounts according to your baby's needs.
- Give extra milk or boiled water as necessary.
- Offer older infants finger foods, such as unsweetened rusks or rice cakes, if they are hungry between meals.

Eating plans for around 6 months

Day 1

Early morning
150ml milk feed

Mid-morning
100ml milk feed

Lunch
Few spoons of baby rice purée
100ml milk feed

Tea-time
Few spoons of banana or apple purée (or combine both once baby is used to each flavour)
100ml milk feed

Bedtime
150ml milk feed

Day 2

Early morning
150ml milk feed

Mid-morning
100ml milk feed

Lunch
Few spoonfuls of potato and/or parsnip purée
100ml milk feed

Tea-time
Few spoonfuls of pear purée
100ml milk feed

Bedtime
150ml milk feed

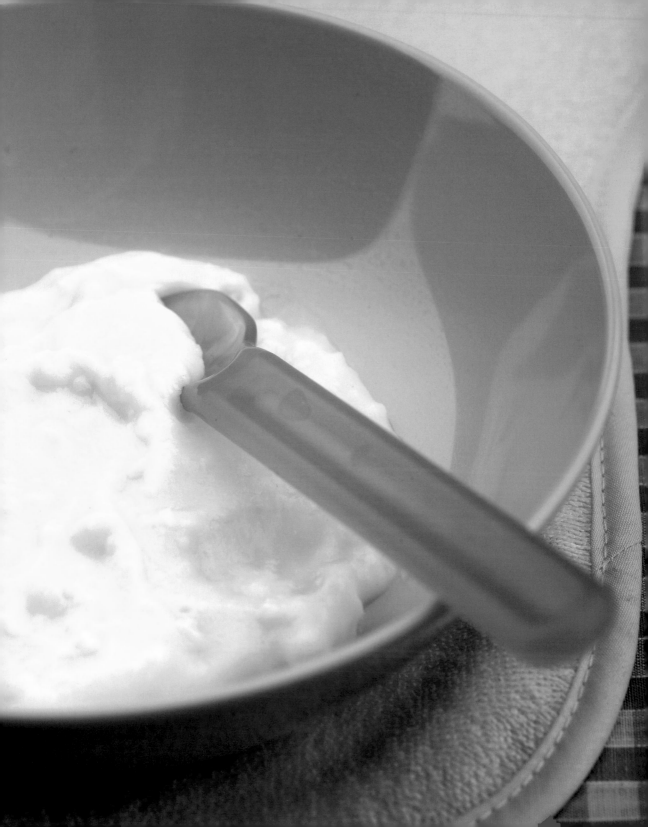

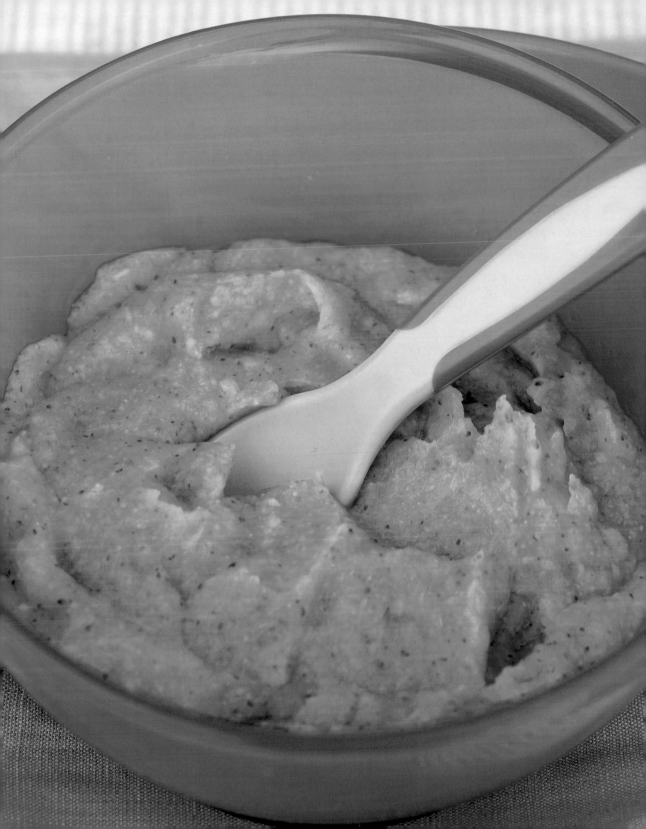

Eating plans for 6–9 months

Day 1

Early morning
150ml milk feed

Breakfast
60–100ml baby porridge
cereal made with breast or
formula milk
100ml milk feed

Mid-morning
100ml milk feed
Unsweetened baby rusk (for
older babies in this group)

Lunch
60ml carrot and red lentil
purée
100ml well-diluted apple
juice

Tea-time
Stewed plum and
bio yoghurt purée
100ml milk feed

Bedtime
150ml milk feed

Day 2

Early morning
150ml milk feed

Breakfast
60–100ml baby rice and
puréed apple
100ml milk feed

Mid-morning
100ml milk feed

Lunch
75ml Cod, Potato and
Cheddar Pie (page 40)
100ml well-diluted apple
juice

Tea-time
60ml broccoli and sweet
potato purée
100ml milk feed

Bedtime
150ml milk feed

Day 3

Early morning
150ml milk feed

Breakfast
60–100ml baby rice
blended with ripe banana
100ml milk feed

Mid-morning
100ml milk feed

Lunch
75ml Beef and Vegetable
Hash (page 43)
100ml milk feed

Tea-time
80–100ml Creamed Pasta
with Vegetables (page 36)
100ml well-diluted grape
juice

Bedtime
150ml milk feed

Eating plans for 9–12 months

Day 1

Early morning
150ml milk feed

Breakfast
60–80ml baby rice cereal
blended with ripe banana
100ml milk feed

Mid-morning
100ml milk feed

Lunch
Beef and Vegetable Hash
(page 43)
100ml milk feed

Tea-time
80–100ml Creamed Pasta
with Vegetables (page 36)
100ml well-diluted grape
juice

Bedtime
150ml milk feed

Day 2

Early morning
150ml milk feed

Breakfast
100ml sieved strawberry
compote with full-fat
fromage frais
100ml milk feed

Mid-morning
100ml milk feed

Lunch
Well-cooked scrambled egg
Fingers of white bread and
butter
100ml well-diluted orange
juice

Tea-time
Tuna and Potato Fishcakes
(page 38) with pea purée
Slices of peeled ripe peach
or nectarine

Bedtime
150ml milk feed

Day 3

Early morning
150ml milk feed

Breakfast
100ml baby porridge topped
with 1 dessertspoon prune
or sultana purée
100ml well-diluted orange
juice

Mid-morning
100ml milk feed

Lunch
Chicken and Mushroom
Pasta (page 42)
Peeled apple slices
100ml milk feed

Tea-time
Red Lentil and Tomato Soup
(page 32)
White bread fingers with
butter
Baby rice with apricot purée
100ml milk feed

Bedtime
150ml milk feed

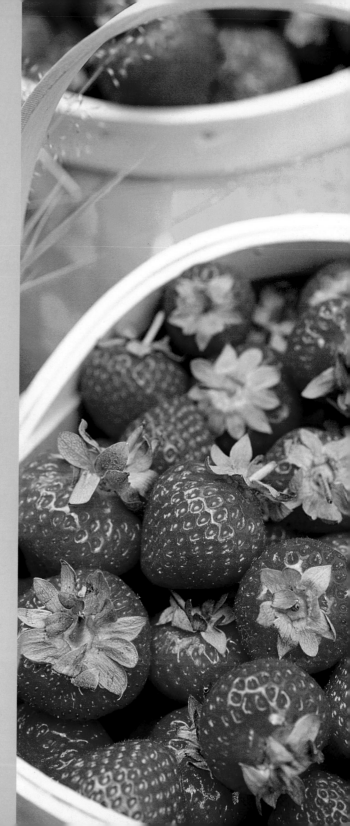

Day 4

Early morning
150ml milk feed

Breakfast
1 Weetabix with mashed banana and milk
100ml well-diluted orange juice

Mid-morning
100ml milk feed

Lunch
Potato and Vegetable Gratin (page 34)
Apple purée
100ml milk feed

Tea-time
Well-scrambled egg
White bread and butter
Peeled peach slices or satsuma segments

Bedtime
150ml milk feed

6 mths+

 12 mths+

 5 years+

Red Lentil and Tomato Soup

This colourful soup is simple but full of flavour. Choose a vegetable stock with no added salt or, better still, make your own (see below). This quantity will serve 2–3 toddlers or older pre-school children.

1 tbsp light olive oil
1 small onion, finely chopped
100g red lentils
150ml unsalted vegetable stock
100ml passata

1 Heat the olive oil in a saucepan and sauté the onion for 10 minutes, or until softened but not coloured.
2 Add the lentils and vegetable stock, bring to a gentle simmer, cover with a lid and cook for 45 minutes, or until the lentils are tender.
3 Add the passata and stir well, allow to cool slightly, then blend the soup thoroughly in an electric blender. Reheat to serve.

4–6 servings

Good source of: protein, complex carbohydrate, carotenoids, potassium, iron

Special diets: suitable for vegetarians including vegans, dairy-free, wheat- and gluten-free, nut- and seed-free

Suitable for freezing

UNSALTED VEGETABLE STOCK
Many stock cubes contain a lot of salt – so, for children, making your own stock is a good option. Simmer 500g total weight of roughly chopped carrot, celery, onion and leek with a few parsley sprigs in 900ml water for 1 hour, then strain and cool. Refrigerate for up to 2 days or freeze.

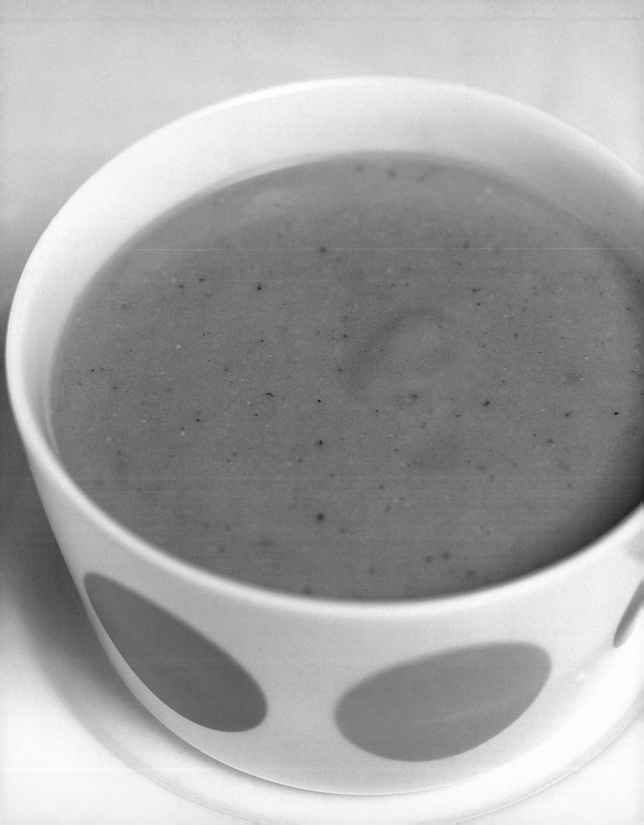

6 mths+

12 mths+

5 years+

Potato and Vegetable Gratin

This is great comfort food for all children, including vegetarians, and contains a wealth of vitamins and minerals. For infants, mash or purée in a blender. This quantity will serve 3–4 toddlers or older pre-school children.

400g waxy potatoes, peeled and cut into large chunks
400g sweet potatoes, peeled and cut into large chunks
200g broccoli, cut into small florets
1 recipe-quantity Cheese Sauce (page 46)
50ml semi-skimmed milk
handful of small rocket leaves (optional)
cooking oil spray
50g Cheddar cheese, grated

1 Preheat the oven to 180°C/gas 4. Parboil the two types of potato until nearly cooked but still firm, drain and cool slightly. Parboil the broccoli florets for 3–4 minutes, then drain. Heat the cheese sauce in a saucepan with the extra milk and then stir in the rocket leaves (if using).
2 Spray a family-sized gratin or baking dish with cooking oil spray. When the potatoes are cool enough to handle, slice them thinly and arrange half in the base of the dish. Pour over half the warm cheese sauce and then arrange the remaining potato in the dish, followed by the broccoli florets and the remaining cheese sauce. Take care to ensure all the pieces of broccoli are covered with some sauce.
3 Sprinkle over the grated cheese and bake for about 25 minutes, or until the top is bubbling and golden.

About 6 servings

Good source of: protein, complex carbohydrates, vitamins A, B2, B12, C, E, carotenoids, potassium, calcium, iron, iodine

Special diets: suitable for vegetarians, nut- and seed-free

Suitable for freezing

of: protein,
ohydrates,
carotenoids, vitamins A, B2,
B3, B12, folate, C, potassium,
calcium, magnesium, iodine

**Special diets: suitable
for vegetarians, nut- and
seed-free**

Suitable for freezing

TIP
Use Parmesan cheese in
a block, not the ready-grated
kind in tubs, which is dry
and tasteless.

35 **Recipes**

Macaroni and Broccoli Cheese

Adding broccoli and tomato to this all-time favourite children's
supper enhances the nutritional value of this dish. Serve with a side
salad or vegetables. For infants, mash or purée in a blender. This
quantity will serve 2–3 toddlers or older pre-school children.

**300g wholewheat macaroni
pinch of salt (optional)
200g broccoli, broken into small florets
1 recipe-quantity Cheese Sauce (page 46)
4 tbsp stale breadcrumbs
25g Parmesan cheese, finely grated (see tip)
1 large tomato, thinly sliced**

1 Preheat the oven to 180°C/gas 4. Cook the macaroni in very
lightly salted boiling water (omit the salt for infants), drain and
tip into a baking dish.
2 While the macaroni is cooking, steam the broccoli until just
tender and drain. Mix the broccoli with the macaroni and then
pour over the cheese sauce, stirring lightly to combine. Mix together
the breadcrumbs and cheese and sprinkle over the top of the dish,
then arrange the tomato slices around the edge.
3 Bake for about 25 minutes until bubbling and golden brown on top.

Mash with
Wash, pee
1 small rip
Pear
fork.
Wash, pee

Creamed Pasta with Vegetables

For babies under 9 months, the finished dish can be lightly
puréed in an electric blender or thoroughly mashed. For toddlers
and pre-school children, the recipe will serve 2–3.

125g dried pasta shapes
75g broccoli, cut into florets
50g podded fresh or frozen peas
20g butter
20g white flour
225ml whole milk
50g Cheddar cheese, grated
2 whole canned tomatoes, drained and chopped

1 Cook the pasta in boiling water for 8 minutes or until tender
but still firm to the bite, then drain. Simmer the broccoli and peas
for 5 minutes or until tender, drain.
2 Melt the butter in a small non-stick pan and stir in the flour to
make a roux (paste). Gradually add the milk, stirring all the time,
until you have a smooth white sauce. Stir in the grated cheese.
3 Stir the pasta, broccoli and peas into the sauce, and finally stir in
the chopped tomatoes. Simmer for a minute or two and serve warm.

About 4 servings

**Good source of: protein,
complex carbohydrates,
vitamins A, B2, B3, B12, C,
potassium, calcium, iodine**

**Special diets: suitable
for vegetarians, nut- and
seed-free**

Suitable for freezing

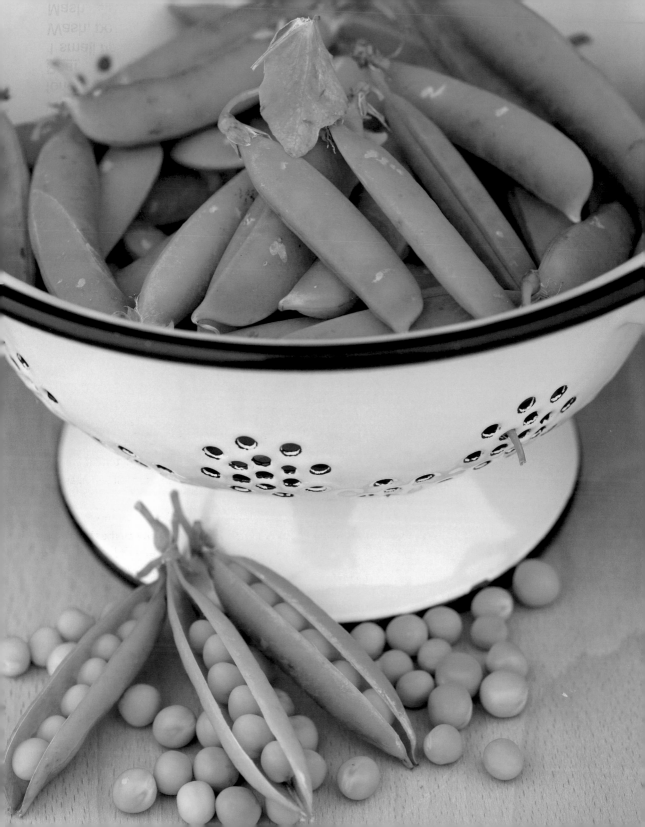

6 mths+

12 mths+

5 years+

Tuna and Potato Fishcakes

You can make these fishcakes with fresh tuna or salmon
if you poach the fish first in water or a water/milk mixture. For
toddlers and pre-school children, this recipe will serve 3-4.

400g old potatoes, peeled and chopped
30g butter
4 tbsp milk
300g tuna canned in water, well drained
2 tsp chopped fresh parsley
1 tbsp light olive oil

1 Cook the potatoes in boiling water until tender, about 15 minutes.
Drain, add the butter and milk and mash well. Stir in the tuna and
parsley, and allow to cool.
2 When the mixture is cool, form it into 8 small patties. (For babies
under 9 months you may need to blend the mixture for a few
seconds before making the patties.)
3 Heat the olive oil in a non-stick frying pan and sauté the fishcakes
over a medium high heat for a few minutes on each side until
golden. Drain on kitchen paper.

4-6 servings

**Good source of: protein,
complex carbohydrates,
vitamins A, B3, B6, B12, D,
potassium, selenium**

**Special diets: wheat- and
gluten-free, nut- and
seed-free**

Suitable for freezing

Do not a[...]
a bland f[...]
Apple
1 small e[...]
Bring 2-4
apple and of: protein,
Apricot B2, B3, B12,
[...]alcium, iodine,
selenium

Special diets: nut- and
seed-free

Suitable for freezing,
but not ideal

6 mths+

12 mths+

5 years+

Fish and Tomato Bake

This cheesy fish bake is a great source of calcium. For toddlers and
pre-school children, this recipe will serve 3–4.

cooking oil spray
450g fillet of cod/coley/haddock, cut into 8 pieces
2 medium-to-large tomatoes (about 100g)
1 recipe-quantity Cheese Sauce (page 46)
4 tbsp stale breadcrumbs
2 tbsp finely grated Cheddar or Parmesan cheese

1 Preheat the oven to 180°C/gas 4. Spray a medium-sized gratin
dish or small roasting tin with oil. Arrange the fish pieces in the
bottom of the dish.

2 Halve one of the tomatoes and deseed it, then chop it into small
pieces and scatter around the fish. Cut the other tomato into thin
slices and set aside.

3 Pour the cheese sauce evenly over the fish, then arrange the
tomato slices over the mixture. Mix together the breadcrumbs
and cheese and scatter over the top.

4 Bake for 20–25 minutes, or until the top is golden and the fish
is cooked through. Serve with new potatoes, or pasta shapes and
a selection of vegetables.

6 mths+

 12 mths+

 5 years+

Cod, Potato and Cheddar Pie

This is a delicious mixture that most babies will enjoy in their first few months of weaning. For toddlers and older pre-school children, this quantity will serve 2–3.

250g potatoes, peeled and chopped
1 small trimmed leek, rinsed and finely chopped
150g cod fillet
200ml whole milk
1 bay leaf
25g butter
40g Cheddar cheese, grated

1 Preheat the oven to 180°C/gas 4 (unless using the microwave). Cook the potatoes in boiling water for 15 minutes or until tender, adding the leek for the last 8 minutes, then drain thoroughly.
2 Put the cod fillet in a frying pan with the milk and bay leaf, bring to a simmer and cook for 8 minutes, or until the fish is cooked through and flakes readily.
3 With a slotted spatula, lift the fish out on to a plate and flake, then mash, being careful to remove any bones which may have been left behind. (For older children you need only flake the fish.)
4 In the frying pan, mash the potato and leek with the butter and cheese and 2 tbsp of the poaching milk. Stir in the fish, then transfer to a small ovenproof (or microwave suitable) dish.
5 Bake for 15 minutes. Alternatively, microwave on medium-high for about 3 minutes and cool to the correct temperature for serving.

4–6 servings

Good source of: protein, complex carbohydrates, vitamins A, B2, B3, B12, D, potassium, calcium, iodine, selenium

Special diets: wheat- and gluten-free, nut- and seed-free

Suitable for freezing

4–6 servings

Good source of: protein, carotenoids, vitamins B3, B6, C, E, potassium, zinc, selenium

Special diets: dairy-free, nut- and seed-free

Suitable for freezing

CHICKEN STOCK

Many stock cubes contain a lot of salt – so, for children, making your own stock is a good option. Simply simmer a chicken carcass with slices of carrot, onion, celery and leek in 900ml water for 1 hour, then strain. Fast boil to reduce the stock and concentrate the flavour if liked. Otherwise, try to find stock cubes labelled 'low in salt'.

Chicken Casserole

A casserole is a good way to introduce a selection of vegetables and these make a contribution to the day's 'five fruit and veg'. Most children like this recipe, which uses convenient skinned chicken thighs and is low in fat. For very young children you can whiz the casserole in a blender. For toddlers and older pre-school children, this quantity will serve 3–4.

1 tbsp light olive oil
1 medium onion, finely chopped
1 medium leek, rinsed, trimmed and sliced
6 skinned chicken thigh fillets, each cut into two
1 level tbsp white flour
125g carrot, peeled and sliced
125g sweet potato, peeled and chopped
1 tsp fresh thyme leaves
300ml chicken stock (see left)

1 If planning to cook the casserole in the oven, preheat oven to 160°C/gas 3. Heat the olive oil in a flameproof casserole and sauté the onion and leek over a medium heat for 10 minutes until softened.
2 Push the vegetables to the sides and add the chicken thigh pieces. Leave them for 2 minutes, without moving, to brown, then turn over with a spatula and brown the other sides.
3 Stir in the flour with a wooden spatula, mixing it in well, then add the carrot, sweet potato and thyme. Gradually stir in the stock and bring to a simmer.
4 Turn the heat down and cook on the hob or in the oven for 1 hour, or until everything is tender and the liquid is moderately thick. Serve with green vegetables and potatoes or rice.

6 mths+

 12 mths+

 5 years+

Chicken and Mushroom Pasta

This is ideal for using up cooked chicken – or simply poach raw chicken fillet in a little stock until cooked through. For toddlers and pre-school children, this recipe will serve 2–3.

125g dried pasta shapes
50g frozen sweetcorn kernels, defrosted
10g butter
2 tsp light olive oil
80g chestnut mushrooms, sliced (or finely chopped for 6–9-month-olds)
1 garlic clove, peeled and very well crushed (optional)
few fresh thyme leaves (optional)
black pepper (optional)
20g white flour
225ml whole milk
125g cooked chicken meat (no skin), cut into small pieces
      (or minced for 6–9-month-olds)

➤ **About 4 servings**

➤ **Good source of: vitamins B2, B3, B6, folate, potassium, selenium**

➤ **Special diets: nut- and seed-free**

➤ **Suitable for freezing, but not ideal**

TIPS
• If serving to babies under 9 months, blend the meal in an electric blender for a few seconds before serving.
• To enhance the appearance of this dish, sprinkle some freshly chopped parsley over the sauce.

1 Cook the pasta shapes in plenty of boiling water for 8 minutes or until just tender, adding the sweetcorn for the last 3 minutes of cooking, then drain.
2 While the pasta is cooking, heat the butter and olive oil in a non-stick frying pan and sauté the mushrooms over a medium heat, adding the garlic, thyme and pepper (if using) after a minute or two. When the mushrooms are just cooked, add the flour to the pan and stir vigorously with a wooden spatula, then gradually add the milk, stirring all the time, until you have a smooth mushroom sauce.
3 Add the cooked chicken pieces, pasta and sweetcorn, and heat through to serve.

- About 4 servings
- Good source of: protein, complex carbohydrates, iron, vitamins A, B3, B6, B12, C, carotenoids, potassium, zinc
- Special diets: dairy-free, wheat- and gluten-free, nut- and seed-free
- Suitable for freezing

TIPS
- For babies aged 6–9 months, purée the mixture in a blender before serving (you may need to add extra water or stock).
- If freezing, freeze the mixture before frying it. To serve defrost thoroughly before frying.
- You can also serve the hash without frying it – just reheat in a microwave after blending.

Beef and Vegetable Hash

For toddlers and pre-school children, this recipe will serve 2–3.

300g potatoes, peeled and chopped
25g butter (or margarine/oil for dairy-free recipe)
50g (dry weight) red lentils
150ml unsalted vegetable stock (page 32)
1½ tbsp light olive oil
1 small onion, finely chopped
125g extra-lean minced beef
1 medium carrot, peeled and finely chopped
1 small tender celery stalk, finely chopped
1 large canned peeled plum tomato, drained and chopped

1 Cook the potatoes in boiling water for 15 minutes or until tender, drain and dry well, then mash with the butter.
2 Meanwhile, simmer the lentils in two-thirds of the stock in a small covered pan until they are tender and the stock has been absorbed, about 30 minutes. Bash the lentils with a fork to mash them a little.
3 While the lentils are cooking, heat half the oil in a non-stick frying pan (with lid) and sauté the onion over medium heat for 10 minutes, until golden. Add the beef, carrot and celery, and cook, stirring, for 5 minutes until the meat is browned. Add the tomato and remaining stock, bring to a simmer, cover and cook for about 20 minutes.
4 Add the lentils and mashed potatoes to the mixture, which should be quite dry, and combine thoroughly.
5 Heat the remaining olive oil in a non-stick frying pan and add the potato and beef mixture, shaping it into a flat cake. Fry until golden on the underside, then turn over and fry on the other side to brown lightly. Allow to cool slightly before serving.

Vegetable Sauce

This is a fairly light sauce, containing small chunks, which is useful in summer with pasta or as a light lasagne filling. For infants, purée the sauce in a blender.

2 tbsp light olive oil
1 large red onion, fairly finely chopped
1 garlic clove, peeled and well crushed
1 large red pepper, deseeded and diced
1 medium courgette, trimmed and diced
1 small aubergine (about 100g), trimmed and diced
100ml unsalted vegetable stock (page 32)
1 recipe-quantity Tomato Sauce (page 47)
few basil leaves, chopped (optional)

1 Heat the olive oil in a non-stick frying pan (with lid) and sauté the onion for about 5 minutes.
2 Add the garlic and red pepper, and sauté for a further 5 minutes, then add the courgette and aubergine and stir for a minute. Add the stock and bring to a simmer, cover with the lid and cook gently for about 20 minutes, or until all the vegetables are soft.
3 Add the tomato sauce and basil if using. Stir well and cook, uncovered, for about 20 minutes or until the sauce has reduced to a nice thick consistency.

About 4 servings

Good source of: carotenoids, vitamins B6, C, E, potassium

Special diets: suitable for vegetarians including vegans, dairy-free, wheat- and gluten-free, nut- and seed-free

Suitable for freezing, but best served fresh

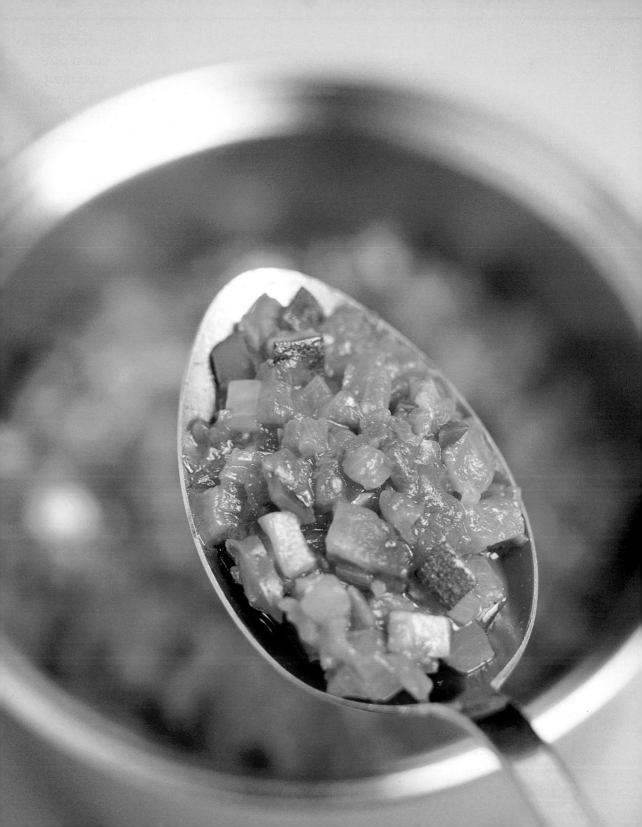

6 mths+

 12 mths+

 5 years+

Cheese Sauce

This sauce can be used in many savoury dishes and is particularly good for children because of its high calcium content. If you replace the cheese with 3 tbsp chopped parsley, you have a delicious low-fat parsley sauce, which is good with all types of fish or ham.

20g unsalted or lightly salted butter
25g plain flour
400ml semi-skimmed milk
1 tsp Dijon mustard
white pepper
75g grated Cheddar cheese

1 Melt the butter in a non-stick saucepan and add the flour. Off the heat, combine with a wooden spoon and then cook over a medium heat for 2 minutes.
2 Gradually pour in the milk, stirring all the time, until you have a smooth sauce. Add the mustard and pepper, and then stir in the grated cheese.

About 4 servings

Good source of: protein, vitamins A, B2, B12, potassium, calcium, iodine

Special diets: suitable for vegetarians, nut- and seed-free

Suitable for freezing

About 4 servings

Good source of: carotenoids, vitamins C, E, potassium

Special diets: suitable for vegetarians including vegans, dairy-free, wheat- and gluten-free, nut- and seed-free

Suitable for freezing

TIP
You could add a little salt for older children, but not for infants and young children.

VARIATIONS
• Add chopped fresh herbs to taste (e.g. basil, thyme, oregano).
• Add extra garlic and sliced black olives for older children to use with pasta.

Tomato Sauce

It is useful to make this sauce in bulk for children as it can be used on its own, with pasta, or as a base for so many recipes, including several in this book.

1 tbsp light olive oil
1 medium onion, finely chopped
1 garlic clove, peeled and well crushed
400g can of good-quality chopped tomatoes
2 tsp sun-dried tomato paste or tomato purée
1 tsp brown sugar
juice of ½ lemon
black pepper

1 Heat the olive oil in a non-stick frying pan (with lid) and sauté the onion for 10 minutes, or until soft and translucent but not turning golden.
2 Add the garlic and stir for a minute, then add the remaining ingredients. Stir well, bring to a simmer, turn the heat down, put the lid on and leave the sauce to cook for 15 minutes.
3 Take the lid off and continue cooking for 15 minutes more, or until the sauce has reduced and is rich and darkened in colour.

47 **Recipes**

The toddler & pre-school child's diet

Once your child starts becoming more active, learning to walk and run, he or she will need plenty of good food to support all the extra energy he or she is using, as well as for growth and development.

Because toddlers have small stomachs and therefore do not have a great capacity for a lot of bulky foods, the type of low-fat, high-fibre diet that is healthy for most adults is not appropriate for them. A high-fibre diet will be difficult for them to digest and cope with, and could mean they may not consume enough calories to provide all the energy they need. A diet relatively high in fat will provide those much needed calories.

Into their second year, toddlers should be managing food similar to that eaten by the rest of the family, chopped up small if necessary – but it is still important to avoid adding extra salt or sugar to their meals. Continue to offer new foods – one or two a week is about right. Children from the age of 2 to 4 years will need a similar diet to toddlers but, as they grow, their calorie needs will increase, along with the need for a little more of many of the nutrients.

A varied and nutritional diet is essential during these early years for proper growth and development. It also helps to shape your child's eating habits for life. For this reason it is important to limit their intake of high-sugar, high-fat foods – sweets, fizzy drinks, biscuits, crisps, etc – that offer little in the way of vital nutrients.

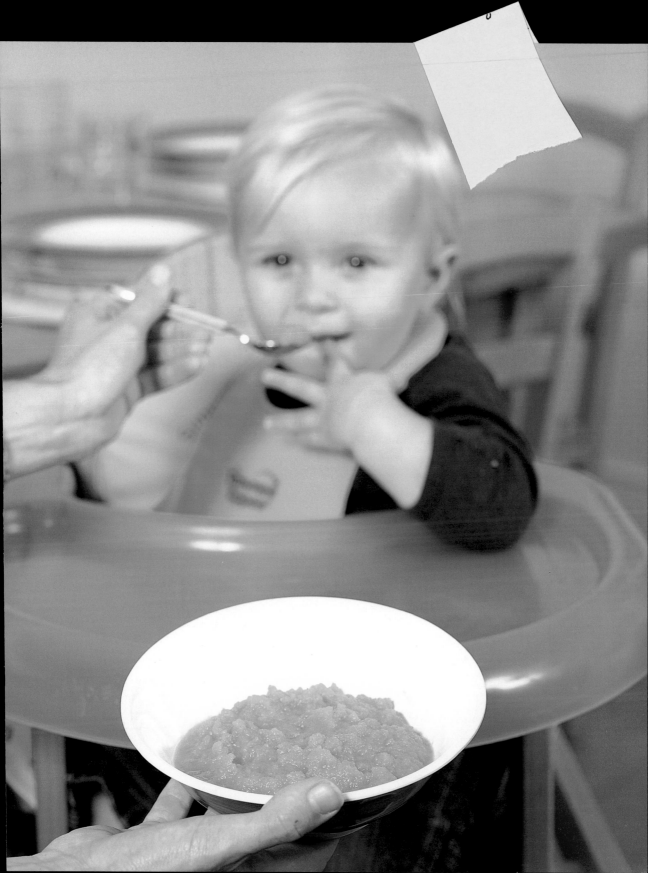

...needs of toddlers and pre-school children

Small children still need a wide range of foods from the four groups: milk and dairy foods; meat, fish, eggs and pulses; cereals, bread and potatoes; fruit and vegetables. They also need enough calories to provide the extra energy needed for growth and increased activity. Fat contains over twice the calories, gram for gram, of either carbohydrates or protein, and a diet containing up to 50% fat is appropriate at this age.

After the age of 1, children can have cows' milk as part of their balanced diet, and whole milk – as well as other dairy produce, eggs and meat – will provide the fat they need. Whole milk and other dairy produce also supply vital vitamin A and calcium, and eggs and meat (as well as pulses and fish) are good nutrient-dense sources of protein. Children under 2 shouldn't normally be given skimmed or semi-skimmed milk as they need the calories and vitamin A that whole milk provides. Children over 1 can be offered all cheese types, including soft and blue cheeses.

It's at this stage parents should be wary of allowing their toddler to eat too many highly processed sweet or savoury 'snack' foods and drinks. Items such as sweets, packet cakes and biscuits, packet desserts, crisps and sugary drinks are the types of foods that provide a high proportion of the salt and sugar in many young children's diets, and research has shown that, on average, small children eat approximately twice as much salt and sugar than is recommended.

As children grow, so their need for calories and essential nutrients increases. Between the ages of 2 and 4 years, the overall percentage of fat in the diet can be gradually reduced from around 50% at weaning, so that by the time your child is 5 years old he or she is getting no more than 35% of their calories as fat. A good rough guide to how many calories your own pre-school child needs is his or her weight in kilos x 100. For example, a toddler aged 2 and weighing 12kg would need around 1,200 calories a day.

By age 2 you can move your child over to semi-skimmed milk if you prefer – this may be a good idea if he or she is slightly heavier than average – but don't start giving them skimmed milk (otherwise they will miss out on fat-soluble vitamins). As your child needs less fat now, it is even more important to keep intake of high-fat snack foods, such as crisps and chocolate, and fatty sugary foods low.

Recommendations for a healthy diet

(The UK Food Standards Agency)

Children should eat:

- A variety of different foods
- A diet rich in starchy foods
- A diet that includes large amounts of fruit and vegetables
- A diet that includes moderate amounts of meat, fish or alternatives, such as eggs, beans and lentils
- Moderate amounts of dairy products
- Small amounts of fatty or sugary foods

Fruit and vegetables

Most of us are probably aware that fruit and vegetables are rich in vitamins, minerals, plant chemicals and fibre, and that the official advice is to eat 5 portions a day – but does this advice apply to small children?

The Food Standards Agency advises that between weaning and 5 years old, you should gradually increase your child's intake of fruits and veg so that by age 5, he or she is getting 'five a day'. I believe that the best way to do this is to offer a wide variety of fruit and vegetables right from the start but to offer them in very small portions, and in plenty of soups, purées and composite dishes.

Then, gradually over these important years, increase portion sizes (1 tbsp, say, at age 2, up to 2 tbsp by age 4) and offer them in more 'adult' form, e.g. sliced, chopped, shredded or whole, as appropriate, so that your child learns to enjoy the natural crunchiness, flavour and form of all the delicious range of fruit and vegetables.

If you hold off for too long it may become harder to get your children to enjoy their 'five', as they do form much of their taste for food in the first couple of years. The eating plans in this chapter give many suggestions for serving fruit and vegetables and there are numerous tips for encouraging your child to eat fruit and veg in the A–Z section. For advice on serving sizes for small children, see 'What is a serving?' (page 53).

See also: Eating Plans p58, Fruit p173, Fussy Eating and Food Refusal p174, Greens p176, Vegetables p212.

Iron

The average iron intake of children in the 1½–2½ age group has been found to be low. Iron-deficiency anaemia may result, which is associated with increased risk of infections, and poor weight gain and development. Make sure to include enough iron-rich foods in the diet, such as lean red meat, pulses, dried fruits, dark leafy green vegetables or fortified breakfast cereals. Adding a vitamin C-rich food (e.g. red pepper, orange) to an iron-rich meal helps to increase iron absorption.

See also: Minerals p185, Vitamins p213.

Salt

Continue to watch your child's salt intake. The Food Standards Agency suggests 2g salt (or 0.8g sodium) a day as a maximum for children aged 1–3 and 3g (1.2g) for children aged 4–6 – much less than most young children eat. Remember when reading food labels, that salt (sodium chloride) is 40% sodium and 60% chloride e.g. a sodium content of 0.4g per 100g food translates to 1g of salt per 100g. (Multiply any sodium content by 2.5 to get the salt content.)

See also: Salt p203.

Drinks

The great majority of your child's liquid intake should still be in the form of milk, water and, if liked, a small amount of diluted fruit or vegetable juices. You should avoid offering your child fizzy drinks and caffeine-rich drinks.

See also: Drinks p153, Milk p184, Teeth & Gums p209, Water p218.

The food pyramid

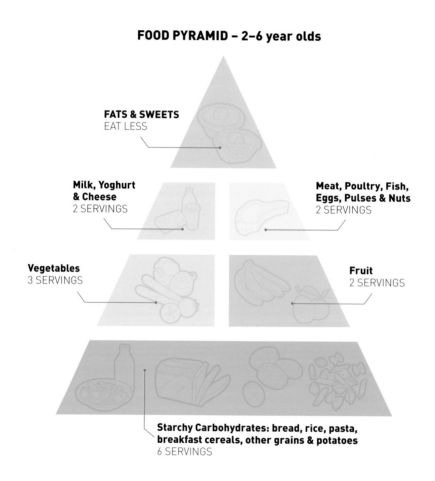

FOOD PYRAMID – 2–6 year olds

FATS & SWEETS
EAT LESS

Milk, Yoghurt & Cheese
2 SERVINGS

Meat, Poultry, Fish, Eggs, Pulses & Nuts
2 SERVINGS

Vegetables
3 SERVINGS

Fruit
2 SERVINGS

Starchy Carbohydrates: bread, rice, pasta, breakfast cereals, other grains & potatoes
6 SERVINGS

The Food Pyramid is a simple guide to providing a healthy balanced diet. It shows you the different types of food children (and adults) need and in what proportions they need them for good health. The Pyramid is suitable for all children, even those who have special needs (for example, vegetarians, vegans or those with food allergies), as there is no need to eat any one particular food, as long as you choose a variety of foods from each group to make up the total recommended servings.

Interpreting the food pyramid

A glance at the food pyramid shows you that the 'base' of your child's diet should be starchy carbohydrates – grains (and foods made from grains) and potatoes. Vegetables and fruits together form the next layer and should make up the next largest part of a child's food intake. Then the 'protein' foods come next – dairy foods, meats, poultry, fish, pulses (including tofu), eggs and nuts. The tip of the pyramid is made up by naturally occurring and added fats and sugars – the foods your child should eat in the smallest quantities.

Recommended number of servings a day are given for all the food groups except fats and sugars, which simply say 'eat less' and should be used sparingly. Actual serving sizes aren't given for the pyramid, but there are guidelines to serving size opposite. At first glance the number of servings may seem quite high but then, if you check the size of what a 'serving' is, you will find it is relatively small.

You don't need to worry about meeting these serving requirements every single day – it is what your child eats over a period of 1–2 weeks that counts. The Eating Plans on pages 58–66 offer guidance on relating the pyramid guidelines to actual meals. The number of servings suggested alongside this pyramid is for a young child (aged 2–6). Older children will need considerably more starchy carbohydrates, an extra 1 or 2 servings each of fruit and vegetables, and possibly an extra serving from either or both of the protein layer groups.

What is a serving?

For an average pre-school child, a serving could be:

Starchy carbohydrates

½ slice of bread

or 2 tbsp breakfast cereal or pasta or rice

or 50g potato (2 small chunks)

Vegetables

1–2 heaped tbsp cooked vegetables

or 2 small broccoli florets

or 1 small carrot

Fruit

1 small whole fruit (e.g. plum)

or ½ larger fruit (e.g. apple, orange, pear)

or 2 tbsp berry fruits

or 6–8 seedless grapes or cherries (stoned)

Milk, yoghurt & cheese

½ cup milk

or 25g hard cheese

or 1 small (125g) pot yoghurt

Meat, poultry, fish, egg, pulses & nuts

30g meat, fish or poultry

or 1 whole egg

or ½ cup cooked pulses

or 20g nuts (a small palmful)

Feeding strategies

Try to match the size of servings to your child's appetite – paradoxically, for poor eaters it is best to offer portions that are slightly smaller than you might think, as you can always offer more. A typical day's eating for a child aged 1–4 should try to include:

Fruit and vegetables 4–5 servings of fresh (or frozen) fruit and vegetables, cooked or raw.
Starchy carbohydrates A serving of starchy carbohydrate food – bread, cereal, potato, rice, etc.– with each meal, in an unadulterated form (e.g. a slice of bread rather than a sticky bun).
Protein 2 servings of meats or alternatives, e.g. lean beef, chicken, fish (avoiding marlin, shark or swordfish), pulses, egg. For safety, still cook the egg well; don't serve children raw or lightly cooked eggs.
Calcium 600ml of milk (whole under 2, semi-skimmed or whole for ages 2–4; alternatively, substitute 25g cheese per 100ml for some of this milk) plus one or two daily snacks/desserts based on yoghurt or fromage frais. For vegan children, calcium-fortified soya milk and soya milk yoghurts and tofu are suitable alternatives.

Vegetarian children

Continue with the advice that appeared on page 13, providing vegetarian children with a good range of non-animal sources of protein, including pulses and dairy products, and ensuring that they don't miss out on essential minerals such as iron, and vitamins such as B12. For further advice, see page 108.

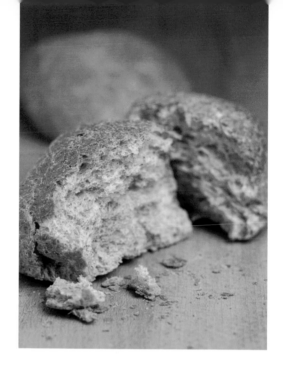

How many meals a day?

Small children often can't face or manage big meals, yet their nutrient needs are high, so 'little and often' is a good maxim.

Breakfast is important and shouldn't be skipped; lunch is a vital refuelling meal for active pre-schoolers and also gives a breathing space in the day, and an early supper/tea is a good time for the family to share a meal. Mid-morning and mid-afternoon are appropriate snack times, as long as these snacks aren't too calorie-rich, while a milk drink and a semi-sweet biscuit at bedtime will help children to sleep.

See also: Eating Plans p58.

Avoid offering sweet and savoury snack foods and drinks as a 'treat', otherwise children may perceive these foods as more desirable than others. Don't ever offer them as a 'reward' for, say, eating their vegetables.

Feeding problems

Experiencing eating problems is a normal and common stage of early development. Toddlers can be notoriously difficult about eating what you want them to eat, when you want them to eat it. The tantrums of the 'terrible twos' can be just as bad at the dining table as they are in your supermarket or at nursery school.

This is partly because children are experimenting with, or being asked to try, new textures and tastes, and partly because they are testing their parents' reactions and seeing what effect their behaviour has. The majority of children will grow out of any problems, but you can help minimize mealtime tantrums and raised stress levels (and that's only in you, the parent!) with the following advice.

See also: Fussy Eating and Food Refusal p174.

Don't worry, stay calm

Almost all children aged around 2–3 have their food favourites and dislike certain foods that they have previously liked, or refuse certain foods just from looking at them, or try a little and then refuse that food next time. Many will use food refusal as a way to get your attention – or a reaction. If they are not underweight and seem healthy, and are eating some foods from each of the groups (see page 13), then you shouldn't worry too much. Getting agitated, or forcing them to eat, will make the situation worse.

Physical causes of refusal

Teething If your child is teething, he or she may feel off-colour, his or her gums will be sore and he or she may be off his or her food. Offer sugar-free rusks or rice cakes to chew on and plenty to drink until the child feels better.
Illness If your child is ill, this may cause them to be off their food. See a doctor and give plenty to drink.
Tiredness and stress If your child is more tired than usual, or worried about anything, such as the arrival of a new child minder, or picking up on the fact that you yourself are troubled, he or she may go off his or her food.

See also: Convalescence p149.

Small range of foods

Small children who will only eat a few different types of food – say, milk, bread, cheese, apples – can be a worry, but seem to do better on such limited diets than you might think. Try to build on a favourite food and work others in. For example, if he or she loves milk, then add a small amount of blended fruit to make a milkshake and gradually increase the amount and variety of fruits used. If your child loves bread, try it toasted, plain, white, brown, with butter, with spread, and then try a tiny bit of peanut butter or mashed banana in a small sandwich. Your community dietitian may advise vitamin and mineral drops – A, C and D are commonly given to small children.

Introducing new foods

Early conditioning Research has shown that if your child has been introduced to a wide range of foods straight from weaning, they are more likely to accept them. Also, delayed weaning (much after 6 months) can cause later faddy eating, as can delay in offering textured foods or chunks of food.

Keep trying The best way to offer children a new food is in very tiny amounts, and you may need to offer it numerous times. Most parents give up on a new food after offering it twice, but it takes 8–10 times for the child to accept the new taste.

Don't mention the 'H' word! Research also shows that children who are told that they must eat up a food because it is 'healthy' or 'good for them' are actually less likely to like or accept the food being offered.

Peanuts and food allergies

Unless your child is at high risk of allergy (i.e. you or they suffer from allergies, asthma or eczema), he or she can have smooth nut butters (e.g. peanut butter) from age 1 onwards – these contain good amounts of protein, as well as essential fats, and are especially useful for vegetarian or vegan children.

Don't ever give whole nuts to children under 5 years of age, as there is quite a considerable risk that they could choke on them.

For high allergy risk children, you are advised to wait until aged 3 or possibly 5 before trying them with peanut products. It is also wise to avoid any foods to which other members of the family may be intolerant, e.g. peanuts (groundnuts) and other nuts, eggs, wheat – or ask your dietitian for further advice.

Small appetite

Be guided by your child's weight. If it is reasonable, then don't worry. Many small children don't have much of an appetite for their main meals because they have filled up on snacks and drinks between meals. A child needs to be hungry to enjoy a meal, so try offering only water or diluted juice for drinks, and snacks of fresh fruit or vegetable batons between meals.

See also: Appetite Loss p136.

A healthy start

Dislike of vegetables If your child only dislikes some vegetables then that isn't likely to be too much of a problem as he or she can get all the nutrients they need from the ones they do enjoy.

Junk foods and snacks By and large, if a young child doesn't have access to these foods he or she won't want them. Sadly, a lot of parents do offer their small children crisps, sweets and so on. At this age you really have control over what your child eats, so don't introduce them. In particular, don't instill the idea that these items are treats or rewards. This is especially important for overweight children and those with a poor appetite.

Sweet tooth Tastes for salty and sweet foods are developed early in life, and although these can be reversed, it is hard to do so when they become entrenched. However, there is nothing wrong with many puddings – like custards, fruit desserts and rice puddings – that can offer a range of important nutrients such as vitamin C, calcium and protein. If your child eats a generally well-balanced diet, the relatively small amounts of sugar in such desserts are acceptable.

See also: Fruit p173, Greens p176, Sugar and Sweeteners p205, Vegetables p212.

Making food enjoyable

Some parents, particularly new ones, worry so much about a good diet for their child that meals become tense and anxious affairs. This can make any small feeding problem worse, as children can easily be put off food by tension – or learn to like the attention that food refusal brings.

Give your child the idea that good food is wonderful, to be enjoyed. Help them develop a love of real food and home cooking. Let them enjoy sitting with you, and other family members if you have them, to savour a good meal and a chat. Even small children can help prepare food – washing fruit or vegetables, mixing, kneading, then taste testing.

If a child really doesn't want his or her meal, never force them to sit there with uneaten food for ages after others have finished. Set a time limit on each meal of 20–30 minutes, and never offer bribes.

Weight control

The number of overweight and obese pre-school children is rocketing, so much so that almost a third of under-fours in the UK are now overweight and 1 in 10 are obese.

These figures are worrying because there are many links between childhood obesity and later health problems. For instance, one study found that children who gained the most weight between ages 1 and 5 had the highest blood pressure in adulthood. Childhood obesity is linked with adult obesity, heart and circulatory diseases, diabetes and insulin resistance, and joint problems.

Most experts consider the overweight triggers to be lack of exercise and too many sweet, fatty, calorie-dense fast foods, snack foods and drinks. Parents should limit these foods rather than feed their children a low-fat, high-fibre, low-calorie type of diet (see page 48 for the reasons). If you follow the healthy feeding principles, recipes, menus and tips in this book, you should be providing your child with a balanced healthy diet that won't make him or her put on too much weight. However, if you think that your child may be overweight, see your doctor, who should refer you to a dietitian for specialist advice.

It is also important that your child isn't undernourished – some children are naturally thin without being short of any nutrients, but if your child is thin and appears to be failing to thrive in any way (pale, listless, lacking in strength or energy), then you should also see your doctor for a referral.

See also: Obesity p189.

Planning your toddler's and pre-school child's meals

For children aged 1–4, the following guidelines apply:

○— Portion sizes for all meals, unless otherwise specified, should generally be guided by your child's appetite.

○— Chop or finely chop any food as necessary for younger children.

○— Provide 2 between-meal snacks if your child is hungry (one mid-morning, one mid-afternoon), choosing from: a handful of dried fruit (e.g. apricots, sultanas), a piece of fresh fruit, a small slice of bread with thinly spread Marmite or peanut butter, a rice cake, a small pot of fromage frais, a breadstick with a little Cheese Dip (page 72), a small chunk of hard cheese (e.g.Cheddar) with a low-salt oatcake or a small slice of Banana Bread (page 101).

○— Provide about 1 litre of fluid a day – half of which should be milk (whole up to aged 2, semi-skimmed aged 2–4), the remainder should be water or up to 2 small cups of fruit juice diluted with an equal quantity of water.

Eating plans for 1–2 years

Day 1

Breakfast
Weetabix with milk
Banana

Lunch
Fish Fingers with Potato Wedges (page 81)
Small portion of peas (lightly mashed)
1 pot of fruit fromage frais

Evening
Baked beans on white toast, topped with
1 tbsp grated hard cheese

1 seedless satsuma

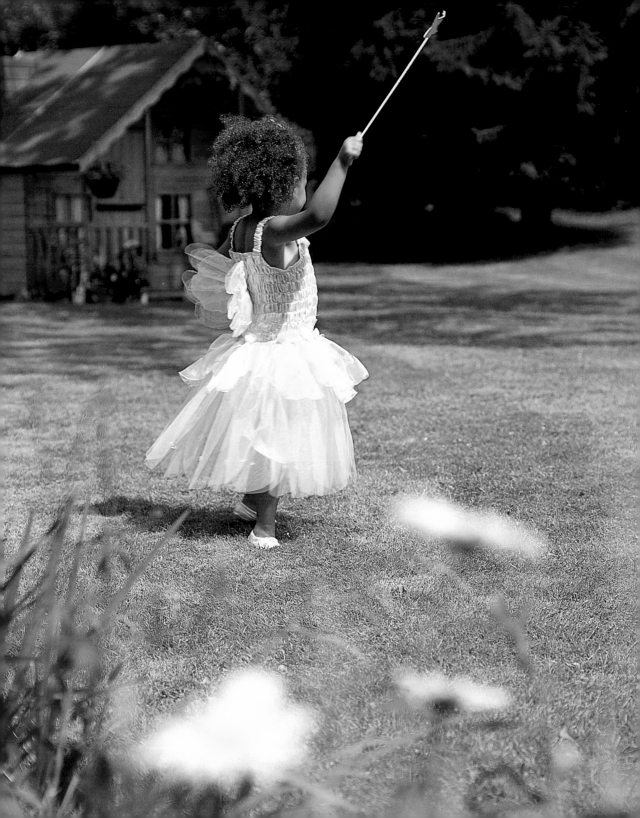

Eating plans for 1–2 years

Day 2

Breakfast
1 medium egg, boiled
Toast soldiers with butter
½ kiwi fruit or pear

Lunch
Chicken Dippers (page 84) and batons of lightly cooked carrot and apple slices, with a mixed light mayonnaise and low-fat bio yoghurt dip, a dash of tomato purée and some lemon juice to taste

Evening
Cooked pasta shapes with Tomato Sauce (page 47)

Day 3

Breakfast
Porridge with milk and a little runny honey
Seedless grapes, halved

Lunch
Beef and Carrot Casserole (page 88)
Mashed potato
Cauliflower

Evening
Peanut butter or ham sandwich
2 cherry tomatoes, quartered
Small pot of fruit yoghurt

Day 4

Breakfast
Small bowlful of Special K with milk and fresh fruit (chopped as necessary)
1 slice of bread or toast with butter and reduced-sugar jam

Lunch
Baked, microwaved or poached white fish (e.g. cod, haddock, coley) served with Cheese Sauce (page 46)
Mashed potato
Broccoli

Evening
Scrambled egg on toast
Seedless satsuma

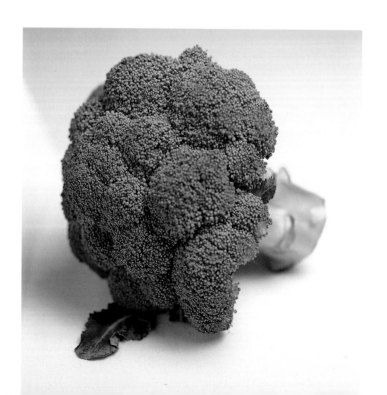

Day 5

Breakfast
Small pot of Greek yoghurt
with runny honey
Apple slices
1 slice of toast with butter
and reduced-sugar jam

Lunch
Plain basmati rice served
with Lentil Ragu (page 92)
Seedless satsuma or pear
slices

Evening
1 small baked potato with
grated Cheddar cheese and
butter
Quartered cherry tomatoes

Day 6

Breakfast
Porridge with milk and
brown sugar
1 banana

Lunch
Cottage Pie made using
Basic Minced Beef (page 89)
Broccoli
½ grilled tomato

Evening
Ready-made pizza fingers
Apple slices

Day 7

Breakfast
Ready Brek with milk
and honey
Seedless satsuma
1 slice of toast with butter
and reduced-sugar jam

Lunch
Roast chicken and gravy
Roast potato
Broccoli and carrot
Apple and custard fool
(apple purée blended with
ready-made custard)

Evening
Tuna sandwich (canned
tuna in water or oil, drained
and mixed with a little
mayonnaise or mayo/bio
yoghurt mix and finely
chopped cucumber
Cherry tomatoes, quartered
Slice of Date Loaf (page 98)

Eating plans for 2–3 years

Day 1

Breakfast
Natural bio yoghurt with runny honey and chopped banana
1 slice of toast with butter and reduced-sugar jam

Lunch
Homemade Burger (page 86)
Potato Wedges (page 81)
Peas
Plum or pineapple slices

Evening
Mini pitta bread filled with Hummus (page 73) and a little chopped salad
Few seedless grapes, halved

Day 2

Breakfast
Banana sandwich on white bread
Glass of apple juice

Lunch
Grilled turkey or vegetable escalope
Grilled tomato quarters
Green beans
Mashed potato

Evening
Boiled egg and bread soldiers
Seedless satsuma

Day 3

Breakfast
Shreddies with milk and chopped apple
1 slice of toast with butter and honey

Lunch
Fish and Tomato Bake (page 39)
Broccoli
Greek yoghurt with stewed dried apricot purée

Evening
Cheese sandwich
Halved cherry tomatoes

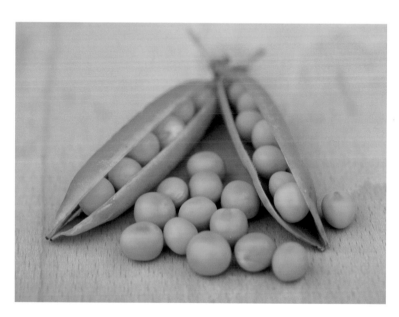

Day 4

Breakfast
Berry and Banana Milkshake
(page 103)
1 slice of toast with butter
and a little Marmite

Lunch
Pasta shapes or chopped
spaghetti served with Basic
Minced Beef (page 89)
Small side salad (e.g. thin
wedges of Iceberg lettuce,
cucumber batons)

Evening
Carrot and Orange Soup
(page 68)
Small soft roll and butter
Small pot of fruit fromage
frais

Day 5

Breakfast
Boiled egg
1 slice of toast with butter
Glass of orange juice

Lunch
Chicken breast slices fried in
a little sunflower oil
1–2 croquette potatoes or
Potato Cakes (page 74)
cooked in the same pan
Sweetcorn kernels
Carrots
Small pot of fruit fromage
frais

Evening
Tuna sandwich (canned
tuna in oil mashed with a
few cooked butter beans
and a little mayonnaise)
Apple slices

Day 6

Breakfast
Weetabix with milk
1 slice of toast with butter
and honey
Seedless satsuma

Lunch
Chunky Vegetable and Bean
Soup (page 69)
Vanilla ice cream with
ready-made fruit coulis and
a few sliced strawberries or
other fruit

Evening
Chicken wrap (cooked
chicken breast mixed with a
little mayonnaise and lemon
juice and some shredded
lettuce in a tortilla-type
wrap), cut into bite-sized
pieces to serve
Slice of Date Loaf (page 98)

Eating plans for 3–4 years

Day 7

Breakfast
Porridge with milk and
brown sugar
Few seedless grapes, halved

Lunch
Roast lamb and gravy
Roast potatoes
Mashed swede
Peas
Banana Split (page 97)

Evening
Cheese Dip (page 72) with
vegetable sticks (e.g. carrot,
courgette, etc.), breadsticks
and apple slices

Day 1

Breakfast
Special K with milk
Chopped berry fruits
1 slice of bread with butter
and reduced-sugar jam

Lunch
Tuna, Pasta and Tomato
Bake (page 80)
Greek yoghurt with stewed
blackcurrants or plums

Evening
Baked beans on toast
Ready-made or homemade
rice pudding with apricot
purée

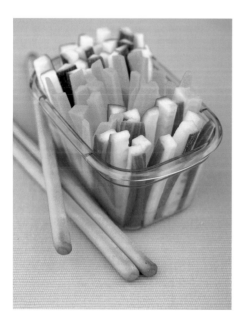

Day 2

Breakfast
Porridge with milk
and honey
Orange segments

Lunch
Chunky Vegetable and Bean
Soup (page 69)
Small soft roll
Pot of fruit fromage frais

Evening
Baked jacket potato, filled
with grated hard cheese
and chopped ham blended
with natural fromage frais
Cherry tomatoes
Lettuce wedges

Day 3

Breakfast
Berry and Banana Milkshake
(page 103)
1 slice of toast with butter
and a little Marmite

Lunch
Salmon and Egg Flan
(page 83)
Cress, tomato and
cucumber salad
Pear slices

Evening
Chicken Soup (page 70)
Soft brown roll
Pot of fruit fromage frais

Day 4

Breakfast
Boiled egg and toast
soldiers
Kiwi fruit or orange slices

Lunch
Reduced-fat good-quality
chipolata sausages
Mashed potato
Baked beans
Seedless grapes

Evening
Cheese Dip (page 72) with
vegetable sticks (e.g. carrot,
courgette, cooked baby
corn) and breadsticks
Slice of Date Loaf (page 98)

Day 5

Breakfast
Apple Smoothie (page 102)
Toast with peanut butter or
soft cheese spread

Lunch
Chicken Casserole (page 41)
Plain basmati rice
Broccoli

Evening
Egg mayonnaise wrap
Seedless satsuma

Day 6

Breakfast
Weetabix with milk
and chopped pear
1 slice of toast with butter
and reduced-sugar jam

Lunch
Fish Fingers (page 81),
or use ready-made
Mashed potato
Peas
Grilled tomato

Evening
Grated Cheddar cheese and
apple chutney sandwich
Fruit yoghurt
Orange slices

Day 7

Breakfast
Greek yoghurt with
honey and berry fruits
or peach slices
1 slice of toast with butter
and a little Marmite

Lunch
Roast beef and gravy
Roast potatoes
Shredded cabbage
Carrots
Fresh Fruit Trifle (page 96)
Evening
Ham and Rice Salad
(page 90)

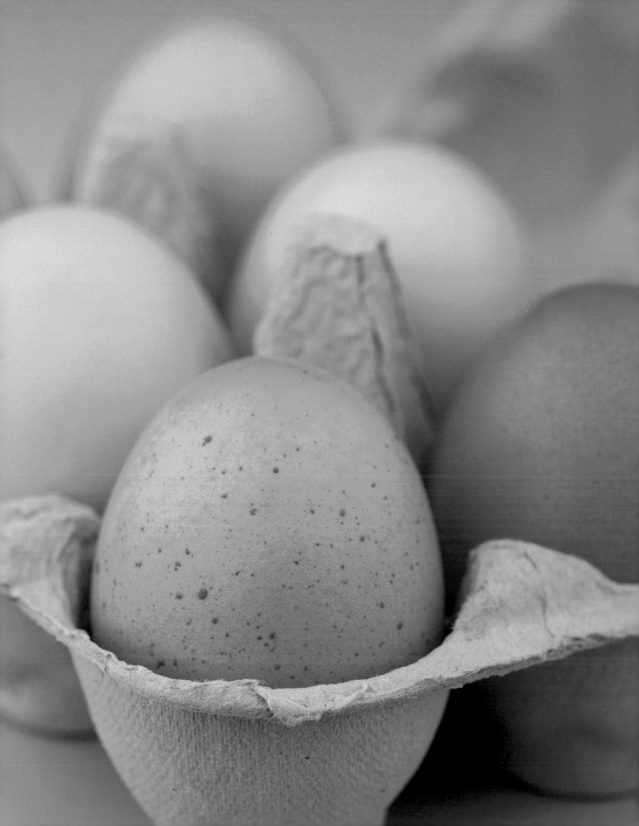

12 mths+

5 years+

Carrot and Orange Soup

This bright soup has an appealing colour and a good, thick consistency which makes it easy for infants and young children to eat, and the tangy yet sweet taste will ensure it is a hit.

1 tbsp groundnut oil
1 medium onion, finely chopped
2 medium carrots, peeled and chopped
250g canned chopped tomatoes
juice of 1 large orange
good pinch of ground cumin seeds
good pinch of ground coriander seeds
400ml unsalted vegetable stock (page 32)
small pinch of salt (as necessary)

1 Heat the oil in a saucepan and sauté the onion over a medium heat for 10 minutes, or until soft but not browned. Add the carrots, stir for a minute, then add the rest of the ingredients, excluding the salt. Stir and bring to a simmer, turn the heat down, cover with a lid and cook for about 30 minutes until the carrots and onion are tender.
2 Allow to cool slightly, then liquidize in an electric blender until smooth. Reheat before serving. Add a tiny amount of salt if required.

4–6 servings

Good source of: vitamins B6, folate, C, E, carotenoids, potassium

Special diets: suitable for vegetarians including vegans, dairy-free, wheat- and gluten-free, nut- and seed-free

Suitable for freezing

TIP
Freeze in individual lidded containers so that portions can be defrosted as required.

4–6 servings

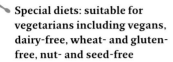 **Good source of: protein, complex carbohydrate, vitamins C, E, potassium, iron**

Special diets: suitable for vegetarians including vegans, dairy-free, wheat- and gluten-free, nut- and seed-free

Suitable for freezing

TIPS

• Small children have not developed a taste for salt so, unless you are serving this soup to older children, just serve it without any added salt.

• For all soups or other dishes with pulses (e.g. lentils, kidney beans) as the main source of protein, serve with a portion of bread – the amino acids in the grain complement those in the pulses to form 'complete protein' (see Protein, page 199).

Chunky Vegetable and Bean Soup

Soups are an excellent way to introduce small children to the varied tastes of pulses. Many children who don't like whole kidney beans will enjoy this partially blended soup, while the small, tender vegetable chunks will help to encourage toddlers to accept 'lumps'.

1 tbsp light olive oil
1 medium red onion, finely chopped
1 medium red pepper, deseeded and cut into 1cm squares
1 (150g) sweet potato, peeled and cut into 1cm chunks
300ml unsalted vegetable stock (page 32)
200g canned tomatoes
200g canned red kidney beans, drained, rinsed and lightly mashed
small pinch of salt (as necessary)

1 Heat the olive oil in a saucepan, add the onion and pepper, and sauté over a medium heat for 10–15 minutes, or until everything is tender and just turning golden.

2 Add the sweet potato and stock, bring to a simmer and cook, covered, for 30 minutes. Stir in the tomatoes and mashed kidney beans, return to a simmer and cook for a further 10 minutes.

3 Allow the soup to cool a little, then ladle half of it into an electric blender and whiz until smooth. Return the puréed soup to the pan, stir well and reheat before serving, adding a pinch of salt if required.

Chicken Soup

Chicken soup has long been regarded as ideal food for anyone who is ill or feeling below par, as it seems to have reviving and restorative powers. Indeed, research shows that chicken soup really does boost the immune system and help speed recovery! It's also very tasty.

2 large chicken leg portions (on the bone)
100g swede or parsnip, peeled and cut into 1cm chunks
2 medium carrots, peeled and cut into 1cm chunks
1 (200g) old potato, peeled and cut into 2cm chunks
1 large leek, trimmed, rinsed and cut into 5mm rounds
2 medium celery stalks, chopped
900ml unsalted vegetable stock (page 32)
1 tbsp chopped fresh parsley
a little black pepper (optional)
small pinch of salt (as necessary)

4–6 servings

Good source of: protein, vitamins B3, B6, C, carotenoids, potassium, zinc, selenium

Special diets: dairy-free, wheat- and gluten-free, nut- and seed-free

Suitable for freezing

TIP
This soup is best served with chunks of bread.

1 Put all the ingredients except the parsley and seasoning, into a large saucepan and bring to the boil, then reduce the heat down to a simmer. Cover and cook for an hour and then remove the chicken portions from the saucepan. Allow to cool slightly.
2 When cool enough to handle, remove and discard the chicken skin. Tear all the flesh off the bones, chop into small pieces and then return it to the soup.
3 Bring the soup back to a simmer and cook gently for 5 minutes, then serve the soup garnished with the parsley, adding a little seasoning if required.

- **About 6 servings**
- **Good source of: carotenoids, potassium**
- **Special diets: suitable for vegetarians including vegans, dairy-free, wheat- and gluten-free, nut- and seed-free**
- **Not suitable for freezing**

TIPS
• You can use slices of beetroot to make crisps, but these are best cooked separately.
• For lower-fat crisps, slice the vegetables very slightly thicker (about 1.5mm), toss them in oil, season and bake on a non-stick heavy-duty baking tray at 190°C/gas 5 for about 30 minutes, turning after 20 minutes. These crisps will not be so 'crispy' and are less suitable for a lunch-box, but ideal for home snacking.

Homemade Vegetable Crisps

Although these vegetable crisps are high in fat, they are very low in saturated and trans fats, and their salt content is very, very much lower than that of commercial potato crisps. They also contain more nutrients.

200g selection of root vegetables (peeled weight)
    e.g. parsnip, sweet potato, swede, potato
sunflower oil or groundnut oil
sea salt
black pepper

1 Slice the vegetables into thin strips using a vegetable peeler or a mandolin. Rinse them and dry them thoroughly using kitchen paper.
2 Heat a 5cm depth of oil in a large saucepan (making sure it comes no higher than halfway up the side). The oil is hot enough when a small cube of stale bread dropped into it turns golden brown within 30 seconds. Fry the vegetables in 3 or 4 batches. When golden, remove with a slotted spatula and drain on kitchen paper.
3 Sprinkle with a little sea salt and pepper, allow to cool, then serve or store in an airtight container.

Cheese Dip

This dip is light but tasty and goes well with raw vegetable sticks, Homemade Vegetable Crisps (page 71) or Potato Wedges (page 81). It can also be used as a toast topper or filling for baked potatoes. By using goats' cheese instead of cream cheese, you reduce the total fat content considerably and boost the protein content.

100ml natural whole-milk bio yoghurt
100g soft rindless goats' cheese
2 tsp tomato ketchup
15g finely grated Cheddar cheese
dash of celery salt

To make, simply blend all the ingredients together in a bowl, cover and chill before serving.

4-6 servings

Good source of: protein, vitamins A, B2, B12, calcium, iodine

Special diets: suitable for vegetarians, wheat- and gluten-free, nut- and seed-free

Not suitable for freezing

4–6 servings

 **Good source of: protein,
complex carbohydrates,
vitamin E, calcium,
magnesium, iron, zinc**

 **Special diets: suitable for
vegetarians including vegans,
dairy-free, wheat- and
gluten-free**

 **Suitable for freezing, or
refrigerate for up to 3 days**

TIP
You can omit the garlic
for younger children. Some
children are allergic to the
sesame seeds in tahini.

Hummus

Hummus is an ideal way to serve pulses to children who might
not otherwise be keen: as a dip, on toast, as a sandwich or pitta
filler, or stirred into soups and stews.

**400g can of chickpeas, drained
juice of 1 lemon
2 tbsp light olive oil
1 tbsp light tahini (sesame seed paste)
1 garlic clove, peeled and well crushed (optional)
salt and black pepper to taste**

Blend all the ingredients together in an electric blender, adding
a little water as necessary. Aim for a soft consistency for dips,
and slightly thicker for sandwiches, etc.

12 mths+

5 years+

Potato Cakes

Straightforward to make, these cakes are a very good, healthy alternative to chips or ordinary mashed potato. They go well with many foods and are especially nice with bacon, ham, eggs, sausage or fish. You can also add chopped-up cooked green vegetables (e.g. cabbage, spinach, sprouts) to the mixture to make a variation of 'bubble and squeak'.

400g old floury potatoes, peeled and cubed
pinch of salt
20g butter
2 tsp finely chopped fresh parsley
black pepper (optional)
splash of semi-skimmed milk
2 level tsp plain flour
1 tbsp light olive oil

1 Cook the potatoes in lightly salted boiling water until tender. Drain and mash with the butter, parsley, seasoning and a little milk as necessary (but keep the mixture firm). Allow to cool.
2 When the mash is cool enough to handle, sprinkle the flour on a clean working surface and, using clean hands, form the potato mixture into 8 or 9 small cakes (be firm, so that the cakes won't disintegrate when you cook them). Dust the cakes in the flour.
3 Heat the olive oil in a non-stick frying pan and, when it is hot, fry the cakes for about 2–3 minutes on each side until golden. With a spatula, remove from the pan on to kitchen paper and serve.

3–4 servings

Good source of: complex carbohydrates, vitamin E, potassium

Special diets: suitable for vegetarians, nut- and seed-free

Suitable for freezing

3–4 servings

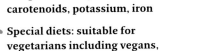 **Good source of: protein, complex carbohydrates, carotenoids, potassium, iron**

Special diets: suitable for vegetarians including vegans, dairy-free, wheat- and gluten-free, nut- and seed-free

Not suitable for freezing

Homemade Baked Beans in Tomato Sauce

Based on canned haricot beans, these beans are quick to prepare, yet they contain far less salt and sugar than canned baked beans. They are great on toast, or with sausages, bacon, ham, baked potato or burgers.

400g can of ready-cooked haricot beans
1 tbsp light olive oil
1 medium onion, finely chopped
1 tsp French mustard
2 tsp soft brown sugar
2 tsp black treacle
juice of ¼ lemon
dash of vegetarian Worcestershire sauce
pinch of salt
1 recipe-quantity Tomato Sauce (page 47)

1 Preheat the oven to 150°C/gas 2. Drain the haricot beans, rinse them and tip them into a casserole dish.
2 Heat the olive oil in a saucepan or frying pan and sauté the onion for 10 minutes, or until soft and just turning golden. Add all the remaining ingredients and stir to combine, bring to a simmer and cook for a few minutes.
3 Pour this sauce over the beans, cover and bake for 1 hour, stirring twice during cooking. If the mixture looks as if it is drying out when you stir, mix in a little hot water or tomato juice. Adjust the seasoning to taste before serving.

Vegetable and Butter Bean Hotpot

This recipe is also good for younger children. Mash the hotpot for children under 1, or purée for those under 9 months. It will provide 4-6 servings for infants, depending on age and appetite.

1 tbsp light olive oil
1 medium onion, finely chopped
1 garlic clove, peeled and well crushed (optional)
1 medium (150g) sweet potato, peeled and cut into small cubes
1 medium (100g) parsnip, peeled and cut into small cubes
80g Savoy cabbage, shredded
200g canned chopped tomatoes
100ml unsalted vegetable stock (page 32)
200g canned butter beans (or cannellini), drained

2-4 servings

Good source of: protein, complex carbohydrates, carotenoids, vitamins B1, B3, folate, E, potassium, iron

Special diets: suitable for vegetarians including vegans, dairy-free, wheat- and gluten-free, nut- and seed-free

Suitable for freezing, but not ideal

TIP
Scatter with grated cheese for extra calcium and calories, though this no longer makes it a vegan meal.

1 Heat the olive oil in a saucepan and sauté the onion for 10 minutes until soft. Add the garlic for the last minute or two, if using.
2 Add the sweet potato and parsnip and stir for a minute or two, then add the remaining ingredients and bring to a simmer. Lower the heat, put the lid on and simmer for about 30 minutes until everything is tender.

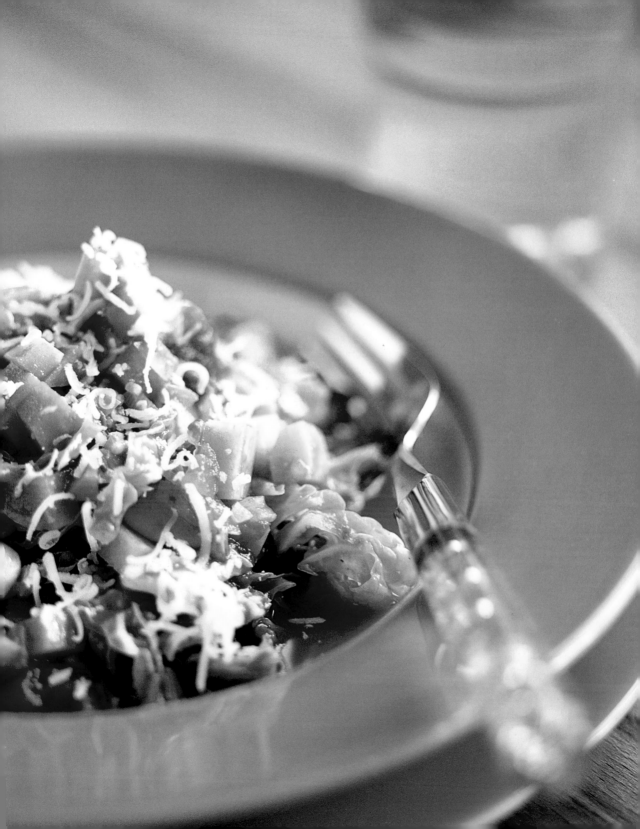

Pasta Shells with Peppers

To increase the protein content here, you can add some grated Parmesan or pieces of mozzarella, or stir in some ricotta, although the dish won't then be suitable for vegans. This recipe is fine for infants – mash thoroughly or purée if you prefer.

1 tbsp light olive oil
1 red onion, thinly sliced
2 yellow peppers, deseeded and thinly sliced
1 garlic clove, peeled and well crushed
1 recipe-quantity Tomato Sauce (page 47)
300g dried wholewheat pasta shells
salt (optional)
16 small cherry tomatoes, halved

1 Heat the olive oil in a non-stick frying pan and sauté the onion and peppers for 10–15 minutes until soft.
2 Add the garlic and sauté for a few minutes more, then stir in the tomato sauce and simmer for another few minutes, adding a little water if the mix begins to look too dry.
3 Meanwhile, cook the pasta in a large pan of boiling water, lightly salted if liked, for 10 minutes or according to the packet instructions, until tender but still firm to the bite, then drain.
4 Stir the cherry tomato halves into the sauce and pour the sauce over the pasta to serve.

About 4 servings

Good source of: complex carbohydrates, carotenoids, vitamin B6, folate, C, E, potassium, iron

Special diets: suitable for vegetarians including vegans, dairy-free, nut- and seed-free

Not suitable for freezing

- About 4 servings
- Good source of: protein, carotenoids, vitamins A, B6, B12, folate, C, E, potassium, calcium
- Special diets: suitable for vegetarians, nut- and seed-free
- Suitable for freezing, before baking

Traditional Pizza

Vary this topping by adding peppers, spinach or artichoke hearts.

225g strong white flour, plus more for dusting
½ tsp salt
½ tsp easy-blend (quick action) yeast
150ml warm water
2 tbsp olive oil, plus more for oiling
200g red onion, thinly sliced
1 garlic clove, peeled and well crushed
1 recipe-quantity Tomato Sauce (page 47)
100g buffalo mozzarella, thinly sliced
1 medium fresh tomato, thinly sliced
2 tbsp grated Parmesan cheese

1 Sift the flour and salt into a bowl, stir in the yeast and make a well in the centre. Slowly pour in the water and half the oil. Mix to a soft dough.
2 Knead the dough on a floured surface for about 10 minutes until smooth and elastic. Put it in an oiled bowl, cover and set aside in a warm place for 1 hour to rise – it should double in size.
3 Meanwhile, make the topping: heat the remaining oil in a non-stick frying pan and sauté the onion for 10 minutes until soft, adding the garlic for the last 2 minutes. Stir in the tomato sauce and cool a little.
4 Preheat the oven to 220°C/gas 7. Knock back the dough and roll out to a circle, 30–35cm in diameter, on a lightly floured surface. Transfer to a lightly oiled baking tray and prick lightly with a fork.
5 Spoon the topping evenly over the pizza, leaving a 1.5cm margin around the edge. Arrange the mozzarella and tomato slices over the pizza and finally sprinkle the grated cheese over the top. Bake for 20 minutes, or until the base is crisp and the topping golden.

Tuna, Pasta and Tomato Bake

To make this dish dairy-free, omit the cheese from the topping and stir the breadcrumbs with 2 tsp light olive oil instead. It is suitable for infants if mashed well or lightly blended and will provide around 5–6 servings depending on age and appetite.

350g dried wholewheat pasta spirals
pinch of salt (optional)
1 recipe-quantity Tomato Sauce (page 47)
400g can of tuna in water, drained
50g Cheddar cheese, finely grated
4 tbsp stale breadcrumbs

1 Preheat the oven to 180°C/gas 4. Cook the pasta in plenty of very lightly salted boiling water (omit the salt for infants) until just tender but still firm to the bite. Drain.
2 Tip the pasta into a medium baking dish. Stir in the tomato sauce and then the tuna. Mix together the cheese and breadcrumbs, and sprinkle over the top. Bake for 20 minutes and serve with a green vegetable or salad.

About 4 servings

Good source of: protein, complex carbohydrates, carotenoids, vitamins B2, B3, B6, B12, C, D, E, potassium, magnesium, selenium

Special diets: nut- and seed-free

Suitable for freezing

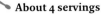 **About 4 servings**

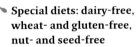 **Good source of: protein, complex carbohydrates, vitamins B3, B6, B12, C, potassium, iodine, selenium**

Special diets: dairy-free, wheat- and gluten-free, nut- and seed-free

Not suitable for freezing

TIP
If cooking the dish for older children, you can add a little sea salt to the oil and potatoes.

Fish Fingers with Potato Wedges

Homemade fish fingers usually contain more fish than commercial varieties and the coating contains far fewer additives. Homemade potato chips are a lower-fat alternative to oven chips. This recipe will serve 2 older children.

400g baking potato (2 small-to-medium potatoes)
1 tbsp light olive oil, plus more for oiling
375g fillets of cod, haddock or coley
50g polenta
1 level tsp fish seasoning
1 large egg, beaten

1 Preheat the oven to 200°C/gas 6. Scrub the potatoes well and halve them lengthways, then cut each half into 6–8 long wedges. Dry them well on kitchen paper and then put into a bowl with the olive oil. Using your hands, coat all the wedges with the oil. Place them on a baking tray, skin sides down, and cook for 30 minutes, or until they are cooked through and the outsides are crisp and golden.
2 While the wedges are cooking, cut the cod fillet into 12–16 finger shapes, taking care that all the bones are removed. Pat them dry on kitchen paper. Combine the polenta with the fish seasoning and sprinkle on to a plate. Dip the fingers into the polenta and then into the beaten egg (in a bowl), then back into the polenta again, then place each finger on an oiled non-stick baking tray.
3 Put the fish fingers into the oven halfway through the potato wedges' cooking time and bake for about 15 minutes. Check a fish finger with the point of a knife to make sure it is cooked all the way through before serving.

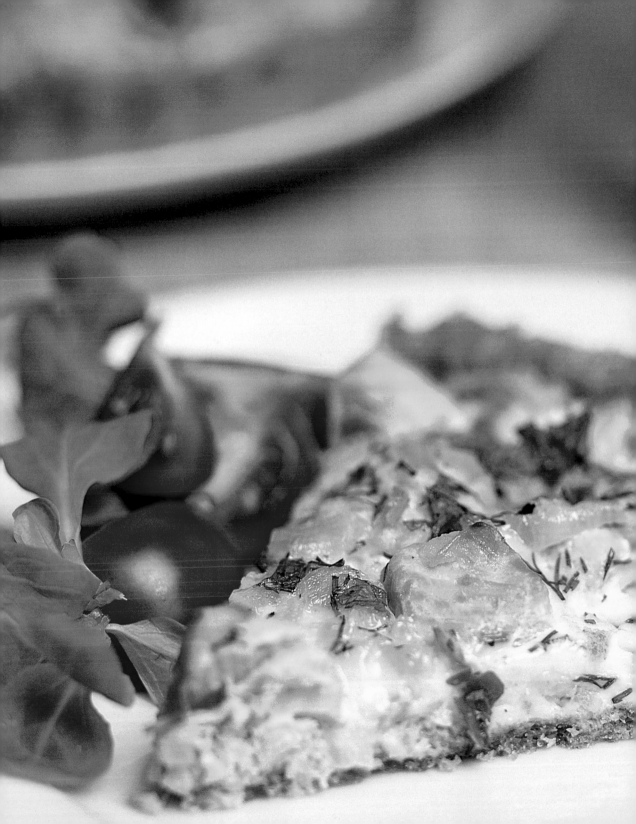

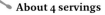 **About 4 servings**

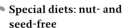 **Good source of: protein, vitamins A, B1, B3, B6, B12, folate, D, E, calcium, iron, magnesium, iodine, selenium**

Special diets: nut- and seed-free

Suitable for freezing, before baking

Salmon and Egg Flan

This flan is a good way of giving children their valuable omega-3s.

225g good-quality ready-made wholemeal pastry, plus flour for dusting
10g butter
2 tsp light olive oil
100g shallots (about 5), finely chopped
200g fresh salmon fillet, preferably organic
2 large eggs
100ml whole milk
squeeze of lemon juice
1 level tsp chopped fresh dill (optional)
1 tbsp chopped fresh parsley
black pepper

1 Preheat the oven to 200°C/gas 6. Roll the pastry out thinly on a floured surface and use it to line a 20cm metal flan tin. Prick the base, line with greaseproof paper and fill with dried beans. Bake for 10 minutes, then remove the beans and bake for another 3 minutes. Allow to cool in the tin. Turn the oven down to 180°C/gas 4.

2 Meanwhile, make the filling: heat the butter and olive oil together in a non-stick frying pan and sauté the shallots for 8 minutes, or until they are translucent and soft but not coloured. Cut the salmon into bite-sized pieces and add to the pan. Stir-fry for about 3 minutes, until the salmon is virtually cooked but still succulent.

3 When the pastry case is cool, tip the salmon and shallot mixture into it and spread evenly over the surface. Beat together the eggs, milk, lemon juice, dill if using, parsley and pepper, and pour over the fish. Bake for 30 minutes, or until the filling is just set and the top lightly browned. Serve warm or cold.

Chicken Dippers

Serve these easy-to-make chicken dippers with a dip, either
of organic tomato ketchup or a mix of equal parts mayonnaise
and bio yoghurt with a little ketchup and lemon juice. Accompany
with baked potatoes or Potato Wedges (page 81) and a mixed
salad for a main meal.

300g skinless chicken breast fillet
50g plain or wholemeal flour
1 tsp sweet paprika
1 tsp chicken seasoning
1½ tbsp light olive oil

1 If baking the dippers, preheat the oven to 200°C/gas 6. Cut the
chicken into strips, each about two bites in size. In a plastic bag, mix
the flour with the paprika and chicken seasoning. Add the chicken
strips and shake to coat well.
2 Now you can either heat the oil in a non-stick frying pan and fry
the chicken dippers over a high heat for about 6 minutes, turning
once, then drain on kitchen paper. Or, alternatively, you can coat
the base of a small non-stick roasting pan with the oil, add the
dippers and turn them to coat with the oil, then bake in the oven for
15 minutes, or until they are golden and cooked through.

2–3 servings

**Good source of: protein,
vitamins B3, B6, potassium,
selenium**

**Special diets: dairy-free,
nut- and seed-free**

Suitable for freezing

- **About 4 servings**
- **Good source of: protein, carotenoids, vitamins B3, B6, folate, E, potassium, iron, magnesium, selenium**
- **Special diets: nut- and seed-free**
- **Suitable for freezing, before baking**

12 mths+

5 years+

Chicken and Vegetable Pie

This pie is a delicious energy-giving dish and a slice will give one portion of the day's 'five fruit and veg'.

1 tbsp light olive oil
1 large leek, rinsed, trimmed and cut into 5mm rounds
350g skinless chicken breast fillet, cut into bite-sized pieces
2 medium carrots (about 150g), peeled and cut into 1cm cubes
50g French beans, halved
50g petit pois
100ml chicken stock (page 41) or vegetable stock (page 32)
1 tbsp white flour, plus more for dusting
100ml hot whole milk, plus a little more for glazing
1 level tbsp chopped fresh parsley
200g good-quality ready-made wholemeal pastry, well chilled

1 Preheat the oven to 200°C/gas 6. Heat the olive oil in a non-stick frying pan and sauté the leek over a medium heat until softened. Add the chicken fillet pieces and sauté until light golden.
2 Meanwhile, cook the carrots, beans and peas in the stock for 3 minutes until cooked but still with a bite. Set aside (don't drain).
3 Add the flour to the chicken and leek and stir well to combine, then pour in the milk gradually, stirring all the time, to thicken.
4 Add the vegetables and stock with the parsley, and stir well to combine. Bring to a simmer and then tip the mixture into a 1 litre pie dish with a pie funnel positioned in the middle. Allow to cool a little.
5 Roll out the pastry on a lightly floured surface to fit the pie. Place on top of the dish, pressing the edges down well and trimming to neaten. Make a small hole in the centre over the pie funnel. Glaze the pastry with the milk and bake for 30 minutes, or until the top is browned.

12 mths+

5 years+

Homemade Burgers

This recipe makes eight small burgers for small children or four 'quarterpounders' for older ones. Serve with Potato Wedges (page 81) or Homemade Baked Beans (page 75), and salad or vegetables, or in wholemeal baps for a quick lunch.

350g extra-lean minced beef
40g stale breadcrumbs
1 level tsp steak seasoning
2 shallots, very finely chopped
1 tbsp chopped fresh parsley
1 medium egg, beaten, or 2 tbsp light mayonnaise
2 tsp light olive oil

1 In a large bowl, combine the mince, breadcrumbs, seasoning, shallots, parsley and egg or mayonnaise. Mix thoroughly then, with clean hands, form into round flat patties on a clean surface.
2 Heat a griddle pan or non-stick frying pan and brush with the olive oil. When very hot, add the burgers and cook for about 5 minutes on each side. Check that the burgers are cooked all the way through before serving.

4–8 servings

Good source of: protein, vitamins B2, B6, B12, potassium, iron, zinc

Special diets: dairy-free, nut- and seed-free

Suitable for freezing, before baking

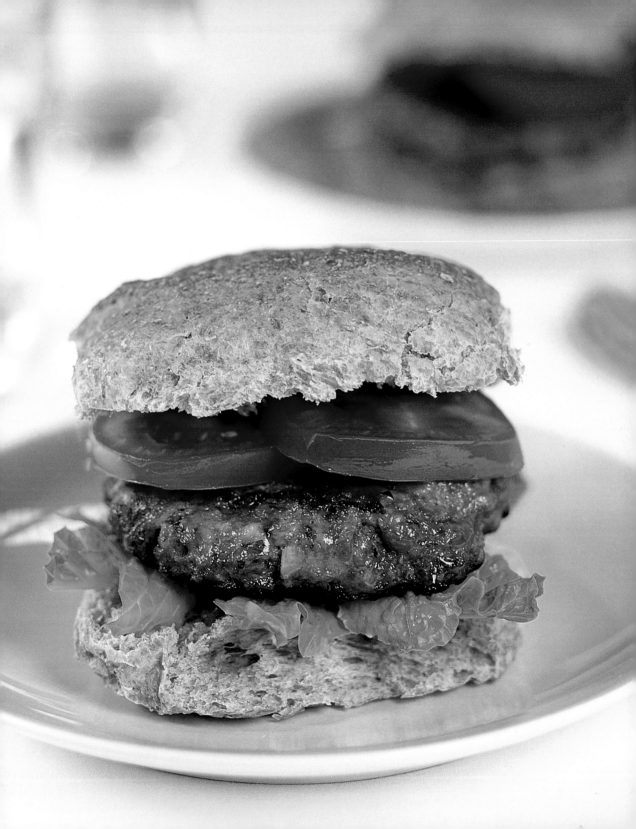

Beef and Carrot Casserole

If serving to younger toddlers, cut the meat and vegetable cubes quite small. For a gluten-free diet, use homemade stock or make sure you buy gluten-free stock. Serve the stew with a leafy green vegetable, such as broccoli, Brussels sprouts or Savoy cabbage.

1 tbsp light olive oil
1 large Spanish onion (about 200g), thinly sliced
1 large garlic clove, peeled and well crushed
350g lean braising steak, cut into small cubes
250g carrots, peeled and cut into small cubes
250g floury potatoes, peeled and cut into small cubes
400g can of chopped tomatoes
about 100ml beef stock (see opposite)
leaves from a few sprigs of fresh thyme
OR 1 level tsp dried thyme
pinch of salt (optional)
black pepper

1 Preheat the oven to 160°C/gas 3. Heat the olive oil in a flameproof casserole and sauté the onion over a medium heat for 10 minutes, or until soft and just turning golden. Add the garlic and stir for a minute, then add the beef and brown, stirring, for a few minutes.
2 Add all the remaining ingredients and stir well to combine. Bring to a simmer on the hob and then transfer to the oven for 1½ hours, checking once or twice to make sure that the casserole isn't too dry – add a little extra stock or water if necessary and stir well before replacing the lid.
3 The casserole is ready to serve when the meat and vegetables are tender and you have a rich sauce.

About 4 servings

Good source of: protein, complex carbohydrate, carotenoids, vitamins B2, B3, B6, B12, C,E, potassium, iron, zinc

Special diets: dairy-free, wheat- and gluten-free, nut- and seed-free

Suitable for freezing

- About 4 servings
- Good source of: protein, carotenoids, vitamins B2, B3, B6, B12, C, E, potassium, iron, zinc
- Special diets: dairy-free, wheat- and gluten-free, nut- and seed-free
- Suitable for freezing

BEEF STOCK

To make your own beef stock, simmer organic beef bones with carrot, onion and celery in water to cover for I hour, then strain. To reduce the stock and concentrate the flavour, boil it for 10 minutes.

COTTAGE PIE

Preheat oven to 200°C/gas 6. Lightly mash 200g organic canned baked beans and mix them into the minced beef mix, then tip into a deep ovenproof dish. Boil 500g old potatoes until tender, about 18 minutes. Drain and mash with a knob of butter, 2 tsp light olive oil, a little semi-skimmed milk and seasoning. Smooth the mash over the top of the mince and bake for 25 minutes or until the top is golden and the mince is piping hot. Serve warm with a selection of green vegetables.

12 mths+

5 years+

Basic Minced Beef

This basic mince can be used for a variety of children's dishes, for example: with spaghetti or other pasta (grate some Parmesan over the top); topped with potato for cottage pie (see left); in lasagne or moussaka; as a stuffing for larger vegetables, such as peppers, aubergines or large tomatoes; or for older children, with added kidney beans, chopped peppers and a little chilli for chilli con carne. It can also be served as it is, with accompanying mashed, boiled or baked potatoes, or couscous and side salad or vegetables.

1 tbsp light olive oil
1 medium onion, very finely chopped
1 medium celery stalk, very finely chopped
300g extra-lean, good-quality minced beef
1 medium carrot, peeled and finely chopped
50g chestnut mushrooms, finely chopped
200g canned chopped tomatoes
150ml gluten-free beef stock (see left) or vegetable stock (page 32)
1 tsp dried mixed herbs
dash of Worcestershire sauce
black pepper

1 Heat the olive oil in a large non-stick frying pan (with lid) and sauté the onion and celery over a medium heat for about 10 minutes until well softened.
2 Add the beef and stir until it is browned all over, then add the remaining ingredients, stir thoroughly to combine and bring to a simmer. Cover with the lid, turn the heat down and cook for 45 minutes, or until everything is tender and you have a rich sauce.

12 mths+

5 years+

Ham and Rice Salad

This tasty combination of sweet and savoury flavours, with the added crunch of wild rice, is popular with most children. Remember that cooked rice should not be stored, even in a cold fridge, for more than 24 hours.

75g (dry weight) mixed white and wild rice
100g extra-lean ham, cut into bite-sized chunks
150g slice cantaloupe melon, cut into bite-sized chunks
75g small broad beans, cooked and drained
50g fresh beansprouts
2 tbsp French dressing
2 tsp chopped fresh mint
2 tsp chopped fresh parsley

1 Cook the rice according to the packet instructions (approximately 18 minutes), then drain and set aside to cool.

2 In a large serving bowl, combine the cooled rice with the ham, melon, broad beans and beansprouts.

3 In a small bowl, whisk the French dressing with the chopped mint and parsley. Drizzle over the salad, toss to mix and serve.

2–3 servings

Good source of: carotenoids, vitamins B1, B3, B6, B12, folate, C, E, potassium

Special diets: dairy-free, wheat- and gluten-free, nut- and seed-free

Not suitable for freezing

VARIATIONS
This salad can be made with bulghar wheat for a change, though it won't then be wheat- and gluten-free. You can also use brown basmati rice instead of the white and wild rice.

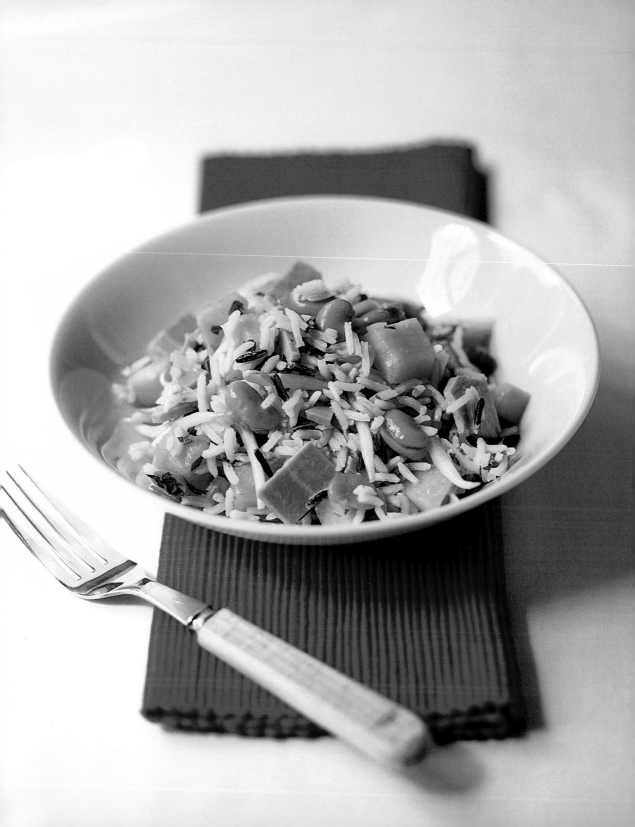

Lentil Ragu

Children often prefer red lentils, but you could use brown or green lentils for this ragu, which would increase the mineral content and provide more B vitamins. It is good with pasta, baked potatoes or rice; it also makes a good vegetarian filling for moussaka or lasagne. If you purée the ragu in a blender until smooth it is ideal for infants.

1½ tbsp olive oil
1 Spanish onion, finely chopped
175g red lentils
1 garlic clove, peeled and well crushed
1 large celery stalk, finely chopped
100g mushrooms, cleaned and finely chopped
1 medium carrot, peeled and finely chopped
100ml low-salt or unsalted vegetable stock (page 32)
1 recipe-quantity Tomato Sauce (page 47)

1 Heat the olive oil in a non-stick frying pan (with lid) and sauté the onion for 10 minutes or until softened and just turning golden.
2 Add the lentils, garlic and vegetables to the frying pan, and stir for a minute or two. Then add the vegetable stock and tomato sauce, stir well and bring to a simmer. Turn the heat down, put the lid on the pan and cook gently over a low heat for 40 minutes, or until you have a rich sauce.

4–6 servings

Good source of: protein, complex carbohydrates, carotenoids, vitamins C, E, potassium, iron

Special diets: suitable for vegetarians including vegans, dairy-free, wheat- and gluten-free, nut- and seed-free

Suitable for freezing

- About 4 servings
- Good source of: protein, complex carbohydrates, vitamins A, B12, folate, C, D, potassium, iodine
- Special diets: suitable for vegetarians; wheat- and gluten-free, nut- and seed-free
- Not suitable for freezing

Spanish Omelette

Most children enjoy eggs, and this classic mix of potatoes, egg and onion is always popular. If you like, you can add a few cooked petit pois to the egg mixture, or add a little thinly sliced red pepper to the onions. Chopped parsley would also be a good addition. Slices of this omelette also make a good lunch-box item for schoolchildren.

400g waxy potatoes, peeled, and halved if large
1 tbsp light olive oil
1 medium onion, thinly sliced
6 medium eggs
pinch of salt
black pepper

1 Boil the potatoes in water until tender, about 18 minutes. Drain and, when cool enough to handle, cut into 5mm slices.
2 Heat the olive oil in a 23cm non-stick heavy-based frying pan and sauté the onion slices over a medium heat for about 10 minutes, or until softened and just turning golden.
3 Beat the eggs in a bowl with 1 tbsp cold water, adding a little seasoning. Tip the potato slices into the frying pan and spread out evenly, then pour the egg mixture over the top.
4 Turn the heat down to medium low and cook the omelette, without touching it, for 5 minutes, or until when you lift the edge with a spatula it looks golden underneath.
5 Meanwhile, heat the grill until very hot. When the underside of the omelette is cooked, flash the pan under the grill to cook and brown the top. Serve warm or cold, cut into wedges.

12 mths+

5 years+

Greek Cheese and Spinach Pie

This pie makes a delicious meal, served with a salad or vegetable.

600g fresh spinach
125g feta cheese
125g cottage cheese or 8%-fat fromage frais or ricotta
pinch of freshly grated nutmeg
2 medium eggs, beaten
black pepper
8 sheets of filo pastry
cooking oil spray
1½ tbsp light olive oil

1 Preheat the oven to 180°C/gas 4. Thoroughly rinse the spinach and put it in a large saucepan with only the water clinging to the leaves. Cover and cook over a medium heat until it is just wilted. Drain well in a sieve, pressing out as much liquid as you can with the back of a wooden spoon, and then pat dry with strong kitchen paper.
2 Beat the two cheeses together in a bowl, then combine with the spinach, nutmeg, beaten eggs and pepper.
3 You need a shallow baking dish just a little smaller than the filo sheets. Spray the base with cooking oil, lay 3 sheets of the filo in the base and brush the top layer with half the olive oil. When the spinach mixture is cool, spread it over the filo and then top the pie with the remaining filo layers and use the last of the olive oil to glaze. With a sharp knife, score the pastry into quarters, so that when it is cooked it will be easy to cut and serve.
4 Bake for 40 minutes, or until the top is crisp and golden. Serve hot or cold.

4 servings

Good source of: protein, carotenoids, vitamins B12, folate, C, E, potassium, calcium

Special diets: suitable for vegetarians, nut- and seed-free

Suitable for freezing, before baking

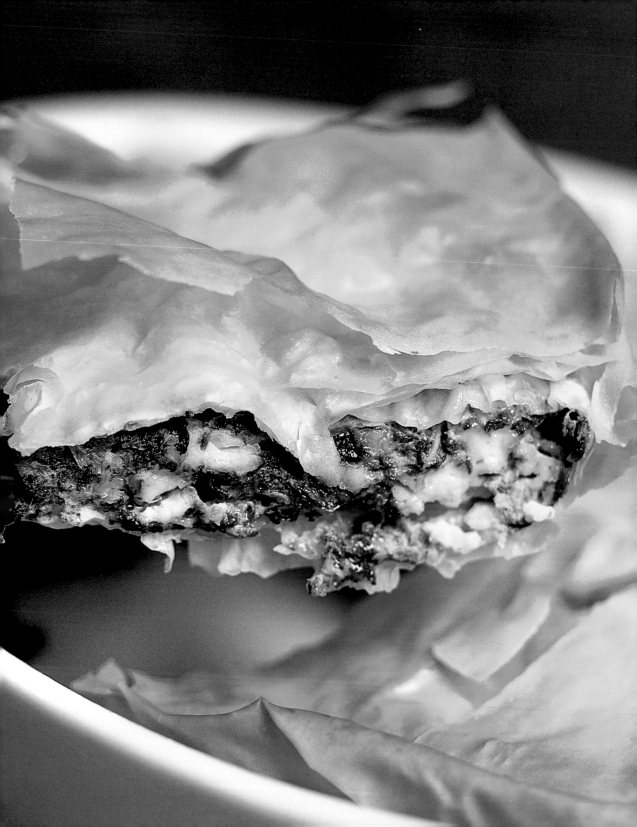

12 mths+

5 years+

- About 4 servings
- Good source of: carotenoids, vitamin C
- Special diets: suitable for vegetarians including vegans, dairy-free, wheat- and gluten-free, nut- and seed-free
- Suitable for freezing, but loses texture

Summer Fruit Compote

This is a rich source of vitamin C and powerful antioxidants.

200g strawberries, sliced
100g blueberries
100g blackcurrants
50g redcurrants
50g sugar

1 Preheat the oven to 170°C/gas 3½. Mix together all the fruits in a baking dish and sprinkle over the sugar and 1–2 tbsp water. Cover and bake for 30 minutes, or until the fruits are tender.
2 Use as a topping for ice cream or yoghurt, with cereal for breakfast, or serve with other fruits.

12 mths+

5 years+

- 4 servings
- Good source of: vitamins B2, B6, folate, potassium, calcium, iodine
- Special diets: suitable for vegetarians, nut- and seed-free
- Not suitable for freezing

Fresh Fruit Trifles

This trifle is relatively low in fat and calories. You can use other berries or chopped canned apricots in juice instead of raspberries.

100g Madeira cake
150g raspberries, plus extra to decorate
1 level tbsp icing or caster sugar
1 large banana, peeled and thinly sliced
150g 8%-fat fromage frais
150g low-fat custard

1 Crumble the Madeira cake into the base of 4 glass dessert dishes.
2 Put the raspberries in a pan with the icing sugar and 1 tbsp water. Warm gently for about 2 minutes, or until the icing sugar is melted and the raspberries yield some juice, then spoon over the cake.
3 Divide the banana slices between the dishes. Beat the fromage frais and custard together until smooth, then spoon evenly over the top of the trifles. Top each trifle with a few raspberries to decorate and chill for 30 minutes before serving.

12 mths+

5 years+

- 2 servings
- Good source of: vitamins A, B2, B12, folate, C, potassium, calcium, iodine
- Special diets: suitable for vegetarians, wheat- and gluten-free, nut- and seed-free
- Not suitable for freezing

Fruit Fool

Higher in fruit and lower in fat and sugar, this is a healthier alternative to commercial fruit yoghurts.

1 large fresh ripe peach
100g raspberries
20g icing sugar
100g Greek yoghurt
100g 8%-fat fromage frais

1 Cut two slices off the peach and reserve. Peel and chop the rest and purée in a blender with the raspberries and half the icing sugar.
2 In a bowl, stir the yoghurt and fromage frais with the remaining icing sugar until smooth. Stir in the fruit mixture and divide between two dishes. Top with the peach slices and chill before serving.

12 mths+

5 years+

- 2 servings
- Good source of: vitamins B2, B6, B12, C, potassium, calcium, iodine
- Special diets: suitable for vegetarians, wheat- and gluten-free, nut- and seed-free
- Not suitable for freezing

Banana Split

This dessert is always popular with children. I like to serve it with a strawberry coulis. To make this, simply purée strawberries in a blender, then pass through a sieve into a bowl to remove the seeds. Sweeten with a little icing sugar and thin with a little water if liked.

2 small bananas, peeled and halved lengthways
100g fresh strawberries
50ml Greek yoghurt
2 scoops of frozen yoghurt
1 tbsp fresh strawberry coulis (see above)

1 Arrange the banana halves in an oblong dish. Chop half of the strawberries quite small and scatter over.
2 Spoon the Greek yoghurt over the top, then add the frozen yoghurt. Halve the remaining strawberries and arrange on top. Finally, drizzle over the strawberry coulis.

Date Loaf

This nice moist, sticky low-fat loaf is also high in fibre. Serve it as it is or spread it with a little butter or spread. It will keep for 3 days in an airtight container.

cooking oil spray
225g self-raising flour
pinch of salt
30g soft brown sugar
75g sultanas
100g semi-dried dates, chopped
30g golden syrup
3 tbsp malt extract
150ml semi-skimmed milk

1 Preheat the oven to 170°C/gas 3½. Spray a 1-litre cake or loaf tin with cooking oil and line with baking parchment. Mix the flour and salt in a bowl, then add the sugar, sultanas and dates, and stir well.
2 Warm the syrup, malt extract and milk in a saucepan until everything is melted. Pour the liquid into the flour mixture and stir thoroughly to combine, adding a little extra milk, if necessary, to achieve a dropping consistency.
3 Turn into the cake tin and bake for 1–1¼ hours, or until a skewer comes out clean. Turn out and leave to cool on a wire rack, then store in an airtight tin or wrap and freeze.

Makes 10 slices

Good source of: potassium, iron, calcium

Special diets: suitable for vegetarians, nut- and seed-free

Suitable for freezing

Makes 12

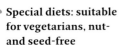

Good source of: vitamin E, calcium

Special diets: suitable for vegetarians, nut- and seed-free

Not suitable for freezing

Apple Muffins

These muffins are deliciously moist and ideal for older children's school lunch-boxes or as an after-school snack. They can be stored in an airtight container for up to 2 days.

125ml semi-skimmed milk
4 tbsp groundnut or sunflower oil
1 large egg
100g soft brown sugar
2 dessert apples
125g self-raising flour
50g wholemeal flour
1 tsp baking powder
1 tsp ground mixed spice

1 Preheat the oven to 180°C/gas 4 and put 12 muffin cases in a muffin tin. In a large bowl, beat the milk, oil, egg and sugar together. Peel, core and very finely chop or grate the apples and add to the milk mixture, stirring well.

2 In another bowl, mix together the two flours, baking powder and spice. Make a well in the centre and gradually add the milk mixture, combining it with the flour.

3 Spoon the muffin mix into the muffin cases and bake for about 20 minutes, until they are golden and risen. Transfer to a wire rack to cool and then store in an airtight tin for up to 2 days.

12 mths+

Carrot Cake

The novelty of baking a cake using vegetables appeals to children, and is a clever way of including them in their diet. If you like, you can make a reasonably low-fat topping for this cake by beating together 225g 8%-fat fromage frais (in which case the recipe isn't dairy-free), a little runny honey and lemon juice. Keep the cake in the fridge if you use a topping.

cooking oil spray
225g wholemeal self-raising flour
1 tsp ground cinnamon
2 medium eggs
4 tbsp runny honey
100g soft brown sugar
100ml groundnut or sunflower oil
225g carrots, peeled and grated
1 tbsp lemon juice

1 Preheat the oven to 180°C/gas 4 and spray a 1-litre loaf tin with cooking oil spray then line it with baking parchment.
2 Sift the flour with the cinnamon into a mixing bowl and add any grains of flour in the sieve to the bowl.
3 In another bowl, beat together the eggs, honey, sugar and oil, then add the carrots followed by the lemon juice. Stir this mixture into the flour until well combined. Spoon into the prepared tin, then smooth the top.
4 Bake for 25 minutes, or until a skewer inserted into the centre comes out clean. Leave to cool in the tin for a few minutes, then remove and place on a wire rack to cool completely. Store in an airtight tin for up to a few days, or wrap and freeze.

Makes 12 slices

Good source of: complex carbohydrates, carotenoids, vitamins B1, B3, B6, magnesium, selenium

Special diets: suitable for vegetarians, dairy-free, nut- and seed-free

Suitable for freezing

- Makes 12 slices
- Good source of: vitamins A, B1, B3, B6, B12, folate, D, E, potassium, magnesium, selenium
- Special diets: suitable for vegetarians, dairy-free, nut- and seed-free
- Suitable for freezing

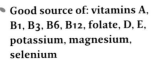

Banana Bread

There are plenty of nutrients in this delicious teabread, which you can wrap and freeze, or keep in an airtight tin for a couple of days.

cooking oil spray
225g wholemeal flour
125g soft brown sugar
pinch of salt
½ tsp ground cinnamon
2 ripe bananas
150ml orange juice
2 medium-to-large eggs, beaten
5 tbsp groundnut or sunflower oil

1 Preheat the oven to 180°C/gas 4 and spray a 1-litre loaf tin with cooking oil spray then line it with baking parchment.
2 In a mixing bowl, combine the flour, sugar, salt and cinnamon. In another bowl, mash the bananas and then combine them with the orange juice, followed by the eggs and oil. Tip the banana mixture into the flour mixture and combine thoroughly.
3 Pour the mixture into the loaf tin and smooth over the top. Bake for 45 minutes, or until a skewer inserted into the centre comes out clean. Leave to cool in the tin for a few minutes, then remove and place on a wire rack to cool completely. Store in an airtight tin – it will keep fresh for several days – or wrap and freeze.

Apple Smoothie

Fruit smoothies made from whole fruit rather than just the juice retain all the plant phytochemicals and are therefore healthier fruit drinks. They are a delicious substitute for milkshakes.

2 ripe kiwi fruit
3 rings of fresh or canned pineapple, chopped
1 Golden Delicious apple
about 100ml apple juice

1 Peel the kiwi fruit, roughly chop and place in a blender with the chopped pineapple.
2 Peel, core and finely chop the apple, then add to the blender with a small amount of the apple juice. Blend to a smooth purée, then add the rest of the apple juice and blend again. If the mix is too thick, add more juice until you get the right consistency. Chill and serve.

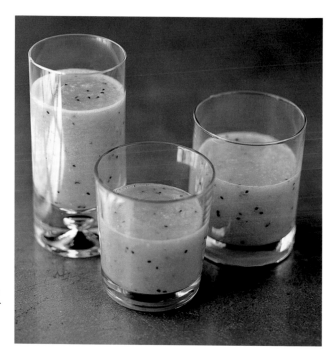

- **2 servings**

- **Good source of: vitamin C, potassium**

- **Special diets: suitable for vegetarians including vegans, dairy-free, wheat- and gluten-free, nut- and seed-free**

- **Not suitable for freezing**

12 mths+

5 years+

- 2 servings
- Good source of: protein, vitamins B2, B12, folate, C, potassium, calcium, iodine
- Special diets: suitable for vegetarians, wheat- and gluten-free
- Not suitable for freezing

Yoghurt Smoothie

This smoothie is naturally sweet and if you use good-quality bio yoghurt, it will help soothe an upset digestive system and restore beneficial gut bacteria after illness or antibiotics. You can also use pineapple (fresh or canned in its own juice) instead of pear.

1 ripe **Comice pear**
125g **raspberries**
300ml **low-fat bio yoghurt**
1–2 tsp **runny honey**

1 Peel, halve and deseed the pear, and cut it into small chunks then place in a blender. Add the raspberries and some of the yoghurt, and blend until smooth.
2 Add the honey with the rest of the yoghurt, and blend again. Chill before serving.

12 mths+

5 years+

- 2 servings
- Good source of: vitamins A, B2, B12, C, potassium, calcium, iodine
- Special diets: suitable for vegetarians, wheat- and gluten-free, nut- and seed-free
- Not suitable for freezing

Berry and Banana Milkshake

This drink is high in vitamins and calcium and makes a healthy, refreshing drink. It is very popular with most youngsters.

1 large ripe **banana**
150g ripe **strawberries**, sliced
300ml **whole milk**

1 Peel the banana, chop it roughly and put into a blender with the strawberries. Whiz to a purée.
2 Add the milk and blend again until the milkshake is thick and frothy. Chill and serve.

Starting school: new influences on diet

By the time children start school, many of the 'toddler' feeding troubles will have vanished. For most parents, having to cope with table tantrums are well in the past. But, of course, there will be new food dilemmas once children reach the primary school years. At this age, children become more independent, are away from home for some meals, and are able to make their own choices about what they eat. Many parents find children begin to demand foods they haven't wanted before, and often these are 'junk foods'.

School lunches are the main meal of the day for many kids, and helping them make wise choices – or going the lunch-pack route – can be a minefield. And, however well you have previously managed a 'no sweets' policy with your young children, competing with peer pressure in the playground can be hard. At home they can be influenced just as much by the power of marketing. On average, primary-age children watch a staggering 2½ hours of television a day, so it's no wonder the many ads for crisps, sweets and fast foods result in a phenomenal level of 'pester power'. These influences – and ways to combat them – are considered in this section. I also look at the growing problem of obesity in young school-children and suggest how to to try to ensure your children maintain a reasonable weight.

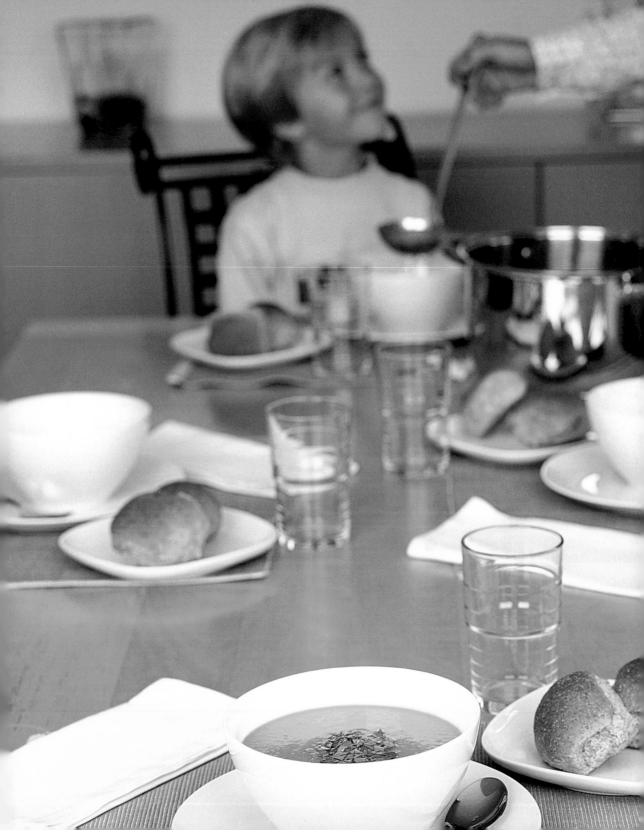

Nutritional needs of primary school children

If you give your child a good varied diet, with plenty of fruit, vegetables, grains, proteins and some fat, you shouldn't really need to worry about exactly how much of each nutrient you are providing. Girls and boys have slightly differing needs. Throughout the primary school years, most boys will need a steadily increasing number of calories – slightly more than girls of the same age – as they are becoming, on average, bigger with greater energy needs.

The more colour on a child's food plate, the more varied and comprehensive the selection of nutrients that plateful is likely to contain – reds, yellows and greens in particular.

At age 5, unless your child has problems such as food allergy or specific health difficulties, he or she can now be given a healthy diet based upon that of an adult, though there are some important considerations at this age.

Here are the main points of difference between the diet of a 5 year old and that of a pre-school child:

Fat The need for a higher proportion of fat in the diet is now over and the level to aim for is about 30–35% of total calories, the same as for adults. For a boy aged 5–6, this is about 67g fat; for a girl of the same age, it is about 60g fat. This means that he or she can use semi-skimmed milk (or even skimmed milk) instead of whole milk. Indeed, as obesity levels in young children are rising, it is wise to keep a careful eye on total fat intake.

It is important to make sure your child has enough of the special health-promoting long-chain omega-3 fatty acids, found in oily fish and some other foods, as the average intake among schoolchildren is low. Adequate intake of these fatty acids in children has been shown to be linked with improved brain power and concentration, and in all age groups with protection against heart disease and other problems.

Nuts Children can now be given whole nuts (unless they have a nut allergy).

Fish Children shouldn't eat marlin, shark or swordfish because of the potential mercury levels in these fish.

Our children, on average, eat a diet that is too high in sodium. Children aged 4–6 should have no more than 3g salt a day in their diet (1.2g sodium).

Fibre Most children benefit from an increased intake of fibre at this age, though many have a shortfall in their diet. You can increase the fibre content of your child's diet by giving them more wholemeal bread, whole grains, pulses and so on. This is particularly important if the child tends to suffer from constipation, and less necessary if he or she is underweight and/or has trouble eating normal child-sized portions.

Nutrients most likely to be in shortfall

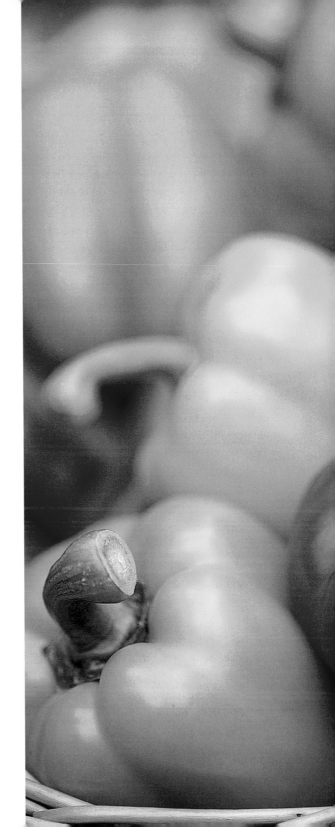

Vitamin A This vitamin has been found to be lacking in a proportion of primary school-age children's diets. Vitamin A is important for healthy vision, eyes, skin and growth. It is found in good amounts in liver, dairy produce and eggs, and it can be manufactured from beta-carotene, found mainly in orange, yellow and red fruits and vegetables such as carrots and peppers.

Zinc This is the only mineral found to be in shortfall in a significant proportion of young children. It is present in good amounts in red meat, dairy produce, whole grains, nuts and seeds. Zinc is essential for normal growth and sexual development, for wound healing and immune strength.

See also: Dietary Fibre p152, Fish p159, Food Allergies p162, Salt p203

The general recommendations regarding diet for primary school children are the same as those for pre-school children:

Recommendations for a healthy diet

(The UK Food Standards Agency)

Children should eat:

- A variety of different foods
- A diet rich in starchy foods
- A diet that includes large amounts of fruit and vegetables
- A diet that includes moderate amounts of meat, fish or alternatives, such as eggs, beans and lentils
- Moderate amounts of dairy products
- Small amounts of fatty or sugary foods

The vegetarian child

The good news for parents of vegetarian children is that the long-term health profile of vegetarians who receive a varied, balanced diet is very good. Several reports have linked vegetarians with lower incidence of cancer and heart disease, and a longer lifespan than that of carnivores. LDL ('bad') cholesterol levels tend to be lower among vegetarians and the intake of several vitamins and selenium are generally higher. However, levels of iron in the blood are often significantly lower in vegetarians than in meat-eaters.

If your child is vegetarian and gets a varied diet (see the Food Pyramid page 52) with plenty of vegetables, fruit and pulses, then you probably have no cause to worry. Dairy produce is a good source of calcium and protein, but should not be relied on too heavily as a substitute for meat, because a high-dairy diet is likely to be high in fats and saturates. However, iron deficiency may be a problem, and you should ensure good sources are included in your child's diet.

Good sources of iron for vegetarians

- dark leafy greens, seaweed
- seeds, nuts, pulses,
- eggs
- pot barley
- baked beans in tomato sauce
- dried fruits
- fortified breakfast cereals
- wholemeal bread
- soya mince and vegeburger mix

See also: Anaemia p135, Minerals p185.

The vegan child

A vegan diet can be very healthy if it contains a wide variety of vegetables, pulses, fruit, nuts and seeds. But a vegan child – eating no dairy produce or eggs, and no meat, poultry or fish – has a greater risk of nutrient deficiencies because the range of foods is restricted. It's important to make sure a vegan child has enough calories and particular attention must be paid to the following needs:

Protein Adequate protein is vital for a growing child but, while animal protein is 'complete', containing all the amino acids necessary for humans, plant proteins (with the exception of soya beans) are not. The best way round this is to offer 'mixed protein' meals that contain all the amino acids needed. This means combining pulses with grains (e.g. beans on toast), or pulses with a starch (e.g. potato and lentil casserole) or nuts with grains (e.g. peanut butter sandwich).

Calcium This is vital for bone development. Good vegan sources of calcium are fortified soya milk, white bread, baked beans, dried figs, leafy green veg, tofu, nuts, muesli, pulses.

Iron Pulses, leafy green veg (e.g. broccoli) and whole grains are all good sources. Absorption from pulses and grains is increased if the meal contains a rich source of vitamin C.

Vitamin B12 Normally found only in animal produce, B12 can be obtained by vegans from sea greens, fortified breakfast cereals, fortified soya milk, Vecon and fortified bread.

Vitamin B2 Vecon, fortified soya milk and fortified breakfast cereals supply this vitamin.

See also: Anaemia p135, Underweight p210.

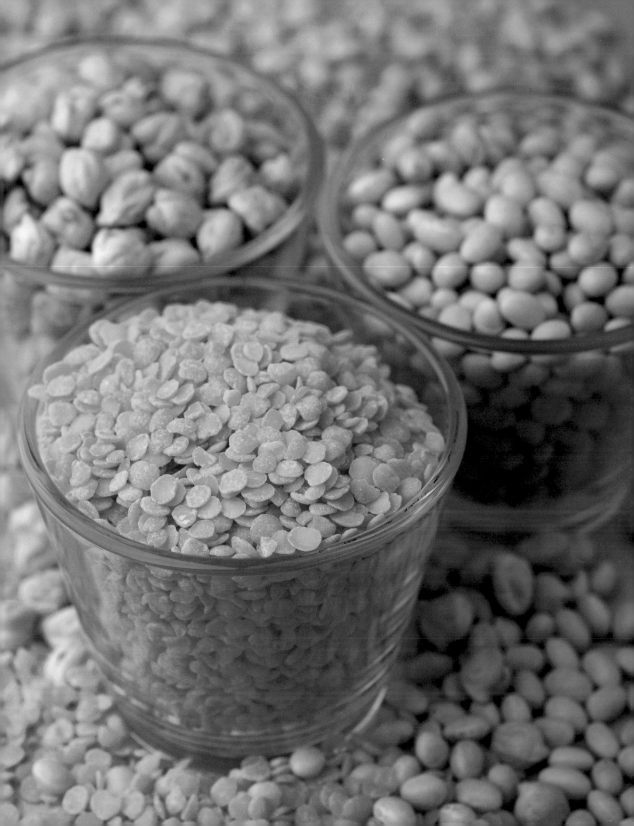

The school day

What your children eat really does have a significant effect upon their intelligence and their ability to concentrate at school, so it makes sense to supply them well with good fuel every day.

The importance of breakfast

If a child eats nothing after supper, their blood sugar levels will be very low by the following morning. If he or she doesn't then eat breakfast, blood sugar will dip dangerously low and this can produce various physical symptoms, such as headache, physical and mental tiredness and dizziness.

Studies have established a strong link between good nutrition early in the day and a child's brain-power. Eating breakfast has been shown to affect the ability to solve problems, and can significantly aid concentration and memory. Other research has found that children who eat breakfast are more creative and have more energy and endurance.

Children who have a good breakfast are much less likely to snack on sugary, fatty foods during the morning, which have implications for health and obesity. Breakfast-time is also an important meal for providing calories for energy and growth, and a wide variety of nutrients. People who skip breakfast are unlikely to make up their daily requirement for some vitamins and minerals, and this is a particular concern for growing children.

On schooldays, few parents have time to cook a full breakfast, but there are numerous cold breakfasts that will provide a good range

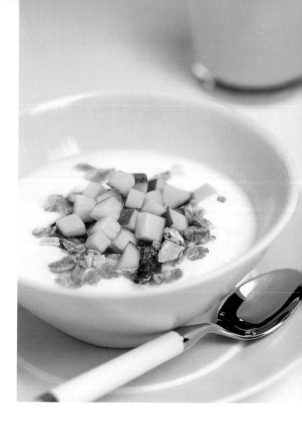

of nutrients and enough calories during the week (see right), while the weekend may be a good opportunity to have something cooked. Avoid cereals and breakfast cereal bars with high levels of sugar and salt.

What is the best breakfast?

A good breakfast for children will include protein, fat and carbohydrate, and will also provide some vitamin C. Protein and fat take longer to digest than carbohydrates and so they will help to keep the child feeling full and keep his or her blood sugar levels even until lunchtime. Carbohydrates are the main fuel for the brain, while vitamin C is vital for the formation of neurotransmitters in the brain and has been shown to be directly linked with increased IQ.

Start the day right...

A good breakfast should offer a high nutrition profile without too much fat, saturated fat, sugar or salt. Here are some suggestions:

- Bowl of no-added-sugar-or-salt luxury muesli with semi-skimmed milk and a portion of fresh fruit chopped over the top OR with a glass of fruit juice (preferably citrus).
- Bowl of porridge made with equal parts semi-skimmed milk and water, sprinkled with a little sugar or honey; slice of white or wholemeal toast with a little butter or spread and some reduced-sugar jam or Marmite; glass of fruit juice or a piece of fresh fruit.
- 1–2 Weetabix with semi-skimmed milk; fruit juice; slice of wholemeal bread with a thin coating of peanut butter.
- Bowl of whole milk or low-fat natural bio yoghurt topped with chopped fresh fruit or berries and a handful of luxury muesli.
- Homemade fruit milkshake (see page 103) and a slice of wholemeal bread with a little spread and Marmite or reduced-sugar jam.
- Homemade fruit smoothie (see pages 102–3) with a small pot of fruit fromage frais and a slice of wholemeal bread with spread.
- Wholemeal bread sandwich filled with a 2 slices of grilled extra-lean back bacon; glass of orange juice or portion of citrus fruit.
- 1 boiled egg; wholemeal bread with a little butter or spread; pink grapefruit segments.
- Low-sugar, low-salt baked beans in tomato sauce on 2 slices of toast with a little butter; orange juice.

See also: Eating Plans p119 for further breakfast ideas.

School lunchtime – packed lunch or canteen meal?

Not all primary schools have a canteen that offers a lunchtime meal, so you may have no choice but to provide your child with a packed lunch, or indeed you may prefer to do so. Both school meals and packed lunches have their plus and minus points – from a convenience angle as well as a health point of view, though a packed lunch may be more expensive.

School meals pros:
- Quicker and easier for you
- Hot meal option especially good in winter
- Basic standards of nutrition mandatory

School meals cons:
- No real control over your child's choices
- Not all school caterers follow good practice – e.g. vegetables cooked early and kept warm lose much of their vitamin content

Packed lunches pros:
- You control what goes in the lunch-box
- You can provide a balanced lunch
- You can organize the whole day's diet for a balance of nutrients

Packed lunches cons:
- Takes time to shop for and prepare
- Many items sold for children's lunch-boxes are, in fact, high in fats/salt/sugar/additives
- Slight risk of food poisoning if the lunch isn't stored in an insulated container and/or if the lunch-box is stored in a hot room

Basic nutritional standards for school meals are set by the government and menus are based upon eating a balance of foods similar to that suggested by the Food Pyramid (see page 52). Many feel that these guidelines do not go far enough, and that a child can still choose an unbalanced meal from the items on offer – for example, choosing a meal of, say, burger and chips but declining the salad and vegetables that are available. It helps if you talk about school lunches with your child and encourage him or her to make good choices, and it also helps if you've already established good eating habits at home.

Perhaps the best advice is to find out exactly how the lunch system works at your child's school before making a decision on whether or not to opt for packed lunches. Ask if the school has a School Nutrition Action Group (SNAG). Ask to see menus, and to visit one lunchtime to see for yourself. Do the salads look fresh and interesting? Are the main courses swimming in fat? What sort of fresh fruit is on offer?

A healthy packed lunch

Try to ensure that your child's packed lunch contains some foods from each of the following groups:

Starches For example, bread or pasta – this should form a large part of the lunch-box.

Protein Lean or medium-fat protein food – either as a sandwich filling or as part of a salad, e.g. cheese, ham, chicken, tuna, egg, peanut butter.

Salad Either as part of a sandwich filling or mixed with protein and starch into a salad (e.g. tuna, pasta and tomato salad), or perhaps carrot or celery crudités, or a small bag of cherry tomatoes.

Fruit The equivalent of 1 piece of fresh fruit, e.g. an apple, satsuma, kiwi fruit or pear. Try to pack things that won't bruise easily. Or make a fruit salad and pack it in a little container with a tight-fitting lid and supply a spoon. If the lunch-box has plenty of salad, you could pack a mini-bag of dried fruits instead. Mini-containers of ready-prepared fruit salad are available from the supermarket chains, but choose fruit in juice and use these only occasionally.

Dairy Yoghurt or a milk drink or fromage frais – these are full of calcium and popular with most children.

Cake A slice of good-quality cake, such as homemade Date Loaf (page 98), or Banana Bread (page 101), or Carrot Cake (page 100).

Drink Water or diluted fruit juices are best. Try to avoid fizzy and caffeinated drinks.

Other items such as crisps, salted nuts, commercial cakes and biscuits are best kept for very occasional use. If you don't pack these items, your child will simply eat what you have packed. Also try to avoid the convenience lunch-box items that are crowding the supermarket shelves, such as instant noodles, brightly coloured dips, cheese and biscuit packs. These are usually full of salt and/or saturated or trans fats, and most contain additives.

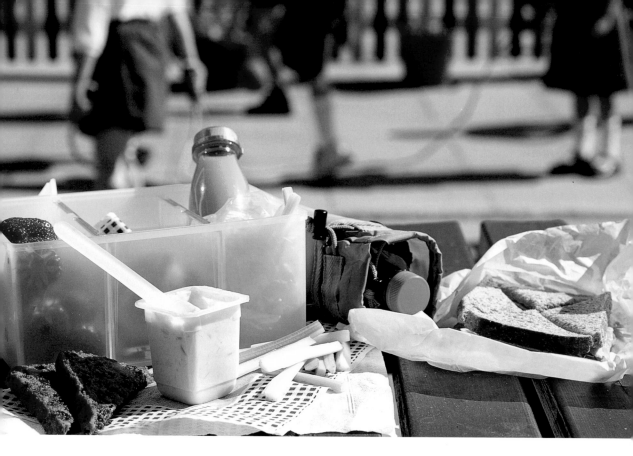

Ensure that the content of daily lunch-boxes doesn't get boring – spend time and use your imagination to provide enough variety of texture, colour and taste. Vary the types of bread used and go for as many different sorts of salad, filling and fruits as you can.

See also: Eating Plans p119, Brain Power p141, Drinks p153, Fats and Oils p157, Obesity p189.

Evening meals after school

After a packed lunch, it's usually a good idea to provide a hot meal in the evening – except perhaps on hot summer days, when a salad may fit the bill. After a school lunch, I would still tend to provide a 'proper' meal in the evening, not just a snack or a sandwich, as,

for the reasons already given, the school lunch may or may not have been nutritionally adequate as the main meal of the day.

On school days it's also best to serve the evening meal no later than around 6pm for younger children – any later and your child's sleep may be disrupted by his or her digestive activity. A late meal may also encourage excessive snacking before dinner, though all children benefit from a small snack when they get in from school – this should be something like a banana, a slice of bread and reduced-sugar jam, a handful of dried apricots, or a pot of yoghurt.

See also: Eating Plans p119, Recipes on p122-9 and p76-95 for ideas for healthy evening meals.

Encouraging healthy eating

What we, and our children, eat is a direct reflection of our lifestyle. In recent years there has been a huge shift away from 'home-cooked' family meals over to fast foods, snacking and eating ready meals.

Most parents of school-age children now work, and working life itself has become increasingly busy, with longer hours, shift work, more stress and long commuter journeys. Many parents haven't the time or energy to direct much thought to how they feed their children. Meanwhile, TV, computers and peer culture exert their influences on children's habits and preferences, often promoting 'junk foods'.

There is little doubt that in order to reverse these negative trends, time and thought is needed at every level, from government down to individual parents. And there are signs that the importance of good food and good diet is being recognized at corporate level. For instance, several supermarket chains have been involved in healthy eating for children initiatives, and the labelling of fresh fruit and vegetables in supermarkets has begun to include cooking and serving suggestions. Even some fast-food outlets are cutting down on the fat in their foods and offering salads and fresh fruit for sale.

The message is that children need to be taught and encouraged to enjoy food in all its variety, and to enjoy cooking – not feel frightened of it. Experts also agree that these ideas need to be instilled at an early age – the primary school years, or even earlier, are ideal.

Parents have a responsibility to educate children about healthy eating, as many bad habits are learnt at an early age. To change these habits you often have to change the whole culture of eating within the family.

This is not all intended to make you, the parent, feel guilty about not having spent enough time or energy on feeding your children or encouraging them to develop their own interest in healthy food. However, it is not too difficult or time-consuming to make a few minor changes that can, overall, have a real effect on the health and well-being of your family.

Get your child to cook and eat with you
Whenever you do cook a simple meal, get your child to help you. From as young as 5, most children are keen to cook, but get little encouragement from their parents. Think of cooking as another 'fun' pastime you can do with them – like playing hide-and-seek or reading a story. Whatever the recipe, there is almost always something your child can do to help, and they will be learning about food at the same time.

What they need to know is that almost all ingredients are good to eat if you know how to go about preparing them. Try to have at least a few 'real' family meals together in any given week, and encourage their interest in 'real' food by taking them with you to markets, looking at cookery books together, planning menus for the week, and so on.

It also helps if you can provide good-quality food in terms of raw materials. The nutritional benefits of organic food may be a subject of debate, but I do find that organic meat, eggs, vegetables and fruit taste better than their mass-market factory cousins.

Healthy meals in no time

These quick and easy meals can be prepared and cooked in less than half an hour.

— Make a quick and easy Vegetable Sauce (page 44) or Tomato Sauce (page 47) to serve with pasta, couscous or baked potatoes.

— Use eggs and cooked potatoes to make a Spanish omelette. Serve with salad and bread.

— Serve egg thread noodles with stir-fried ready-sliced chicken or turkey and a pack of ready-shredded stir-fry vegetables.

— Cook some rice, adding petit pois halfway through, and steam salmon or undyed smoked haddock fillet over the top of the pan. Flake the salmon and stir it through the rice with chopped tomato and cucumber.

— Of course, not all good food for kids has to be cooked. You can serve simple salads with canned tuna or sardines, chicken or lean ham.

Batch cooking

Batch cooking is an ideal way to cook for a family. When you do have some spare time – perhaps a wet Sunday afternoon or winter's evening – make up large quantities of pasta sauces, soups, casseroles and basic mince, and freeze them in individual portions and/or in family-sized portions.

Convenience foods

There is nothing wrong with feeding your children convenience foods occasionally, it is the overall balance of the diet that you need to watch, because a diet too reliant on fried, fast, convenience, junk-type foods is also likely to be too high in fat, saturated fat, sugar, salt and calories.

Many parents say to me that their children 'just won't eat' anything except chips, burgers and so on, and that they hate fresh vegetables, salads and fruit. Research shows that children who are given a variety of fresh foods from an early age continue to accept, and like, these foods – so start as you mean to go on.

I have also found children who do like decent food but their parents just can't cook – over-boiled veg and overcooked roasts are never appetizing whatever your age.

The nutritional profile of many fast-food type meals can be improved with the addition of a side salad or a fruit dessert, or with a good-quality drink such as a fruit smoothie. These won't take away fat, sugar or salt from a meal, but they will help your child towards 5 portions of fruit and vegetables a day.

'Better' convenience food

If you need to choose convenience foods, try to bear these points in mind:

— Buy the best quality you can afford. With food, as with much else, you get what you pay for. Premium-quality beefburgers made from organic meat, for example, will make you feel better about feeding burgers to your child.

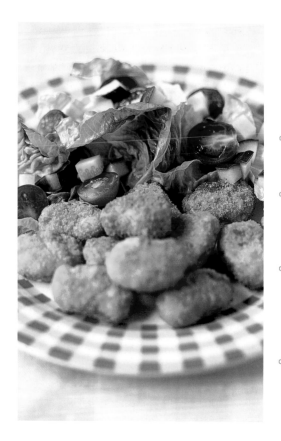

Add fresh fruit and salads to ready meals, like chicken nuggets, fish fingers, burgers, etc.

Make your own cakes or buy them from your local farmers' market or Women's Institute, rather than those that come packaged with long lists of additives.

Buy frozen or chilled counter items rather cans or packets (e.g. soups), which usually have more additives. Chilled counter items are also likely to have a better nutritional profile.

See also: Fruit p173, Fussy Eating and Food Refusal p174, Vegetables p212.

Alternatives to 'junk foods'

As drinks and snacks and foods such as colas, crisps and sweets now account for a large percentage of school-age children's total diet, it makes sense to find ways to reduce their consumption:

Make sure your child has breakfast, so that they won't need be tempted by the school vending machine if there is one.

When they get home from school (and in other between-meal situations), ensure there is bread and honey or bananas for a quick starchy snack.

If he or she is out with friends, pop a pack of fresh shelled nuts or dried fruit in a pocket as well as a bottle of still or fizzy water in their bag. Make sure they have a nutritious meal/snack before they go.

Remember what you don't buy, your children can't eat.

If your child has got out of the habit of eating decently, the best way to get him or her to eat more healthily is by stealth. At first, add chopped vegetables to casseroles, include diced veg in mince mixtures and burgers, and purée them in soups. Purée fruits and serve them stirred into yoghurt or custard.

Pester power

Don't feel angry with your child if he or she pesters you for a food or drink you'd rather they didn't have. They are being influenced via TV ads, via packaging, via special offers and free gifts, by linking up with favourite characters from books or TV; via sponsorship of sports events – even by sponsorship of school products and school events. Bright coloured packaging adds to the appeal – even the food itself may be bright with artificial additives. Around 75% of foods marketed to children contain high levels of fats, sugars and/or salt, and may be described as nutritionally poor.

But you do have to exercise your right to say 'no' to a child's demands. After all, you hold the purse strings. Though it may be easy and convenient to give in to your child's demands, the short-term relief can never outweigh the long-term negative health effects of a poor diet.

Sweets – to ban or limit?

⚬ First, limit – bans rarely work and only make the child feel guilty or resentful.

⚬ Secondly, when you do allow your child chocolate or sweets, make sure they are good-quality.

⚬ Thirdly – sweets are better given to your child at the end of a meal rather than as a between-meal snack.

⚬ Fourthly – never offer sweets as a reward or bribe.

⚬ Finally – all children seem to like a sweet taste, so remember that fresh and dried fruits are high in natural sugar and make a good alternative with added nutrient value.

See also: Fried Food p172, Ready Meals p202.

Weight issues

Overweight and obesity levels are soaring in primary school-age children across much of the world, not least in the UK. In the UK, for example, 20% of 6-year-olds are overweight and 10% are obese, according to a report from the Association for the Study of Obesity.

Childhood overweight is linked with a sedentary lifestyle and a decline in sports participation, and an increase in consumption of fatty, sugary foods and drinks. For instance, children in the UK eat 25 times as many sweets and drink 30 times as many soft drinks as they did 50 years ago.

One study has found that consumption of sugary drinks is directly linked with obesity. Another has linked obesity with the increase in portion sizes, particularly of fast foods. Meanwhile, many children take little exercise. Far fewer children now walk to school and many do less than half an hour of 'moderate' exercise a day (which includes walking around in the home and school). Most children do little in the way of heart-healthy, calorie-burning aerobic exercise, as sports participation in school has decreased. On the other hand, children watch more and more television or play computer games.

Obesity is having serious repercussions on child health – and later adult health – with childhood incidence of high cholesterol, high blood pressure and insulin resistance, which is an early sign of type-2 diabetes.

Weight control

Prevention is definitely better than cure – and a general healthy diet which follows the principles of the Food Pyramid (see pages 52–3), plus regular exercise, should ensure that your child doesn't become overweight.

If a child is already overweight, however, experts advise that the best method of dealing with this is to try to maintain the current weight while the child grows. That is, you don't put the child on a diet to lose weight, but as they get taller they will gradually 'grow into' their weight and slim down. For more information of practical ways to achieve this, see Obesity (page 189). The strategies outlined there should be enough to reduce an overweight child's calorie intake sufficiently. You might also visit your doctor and ask to see your local dietitian.

Exercise

Try to encourage your child to take at least an hour's proper exercise a day:

- Make the exercise something they will enjoy – for example, take them swimming or cycling.
- Give walks a purpose, such as feeding the ducks, bird-watching, car-spotting or orienteering, so children don't become bored.
- Encourage him or her to join a sports club, e.g. football or cricket, for children who like team games, or a gymnastics or athletics club for others.
- If possible, try to walk your child to where you have to go rather than taking the car.

- In summer, encourage ball games in the park or garden and put a time limit on indoor activities such as TV or computer games.

Be diplomatic

There is evidence that even young children can become over-worried about their weight. Some lose a great deal of confidence if their parents make them feel fat. So try to keep weight control a low-key issue. There's no need for them to feel hungry or deprived, just concentrate on all the foods he or she can eat, rather than on the ones they should cut down on. It's preferable to avoid the 'diet' word and don't weigh your child regularly. Lead by example – eat healthily yourself and show a positive attitude.

See also: Fats and Oils p157, Obesity p189, Sugar and Sweeteners p205.

Planning your primary school child's meals

For portion sizes, be guided by your child's appetite and/or need to control weight.

⚬ Allow at least 300ml semi-skimmed (or skimmed) milk a day for use as a drink. Ideally the remainder of the drinks should be water or fruit juice diluted with water. Total fluid intake should be around 1–1.5 litres.

⚬ If a child has a school canteen lunch, ask what he or she has eaten and offer guidance on what to choose. The school meals listed here are sample 'healthier' choices.

⚬ Vegetarians can substitute meat or fish meals with vegetarian options from the recipe sections, such as Pasta with Vegetable Sauce (page 44), Pasta Shells with Peppers (page 78), Macaroni and Broccoli Cheese (page 35), Baked Eggs and Peppers (page 125), Greek Cheese and Spinach Pie (page 94), Traditional Pizza (page 79) or Vegetable Burgers (page 126). Recipes suitable for vegans are indicated in the recipe sections.

⚬ Suitable vegetarian packed lunches include any bread, roll or pitta with plenty of salad and either cheese, egg, vegetable pâté, Hummus (page 73) or cooked vegetarian sausage; a salad based on cooked pasta or rice with chopped egg, cheese or tofu, chopped salad items, nuts, seeds, dried fruits; or a flask of homemade soup; or a bean or cheese dip, such as Hummus (page 73) or Cheese Dip (page 72) with crudités and breadsticks.

Eating plans for 5–6 years

Monday

Breakfast
Weetabix with milk
Banana

Packed school lunch
Peanut butter sandwich on wholemeal bread
Satsuma
Slice of Carrot Cake (page 100)
Small pot of fromage frais

Late-afternoon snack
Slice of bread and honey
A handful of sultanas

Evening
Chicken and Pasta Salad (page 124)
Spring greens or runner beans
Fruit Fool (page 97)

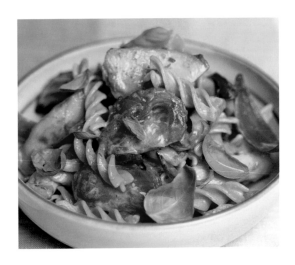

Eating plans for 5–6 years

Tuesday

Breakfast
Toast with a little butter
and reduced-sugar jam
Kiwi fruit
Small pot of fromage frais

School cafeteria lunch
Vegeburger or beefburger
in a bun
Side salad
Banana

Afternoon snack
Slice of Date Loaf (page 98)
Handful of dried apricots

Evening
Pasta with Vegetable Sauce
(page 44)
Summer Fruit Compote
(page 96)
Ice cream

Wednesday

Breakfast
Real porridge made with
semi-skimmed milk with
a handful of raisins added
Orange juice

Packed lunch
Tuna (canned in water)
and sliced tomato sandwich
on wholemeal bread
Slice of Banana Bread
(page 101)
Apple
Fruit yoghurt

Afternoon snack
Pear
Low-salt cracker with a
small piece of Cheddar
cheese

Evening
Spanish Omelette (page 93)
Crusty bread
Salad

Thursday

Breakfast
Special K with fruit pieces
Semi-skimmed milk
Peach or plum

School cafeteria lunch
Cheese and tomato pizza
Side salad
Fruit yoghurt

Afternoon snack
Apple and satsuma
segments with natural
fromage frais used as dip

Evening
Chicken and Vegetable Pie
(page 85)
Spring greens
New potatoes

Friday

Breakfast
Luxury muesli with
semi-skimmed milk
Berry fruits

Packed lunch
White bap filled with lean
ham and chopped salad
Small bag of Homemade
Vegetable Crisps (page 71)
Fruit fromage frais
Satsuma

Afternoon snack
Banana and a handful
of sultanas

Evening
Tuna, Pasta and Tomato
Bake (page 80)
Broccoli or green salad

Saturday

Breakfast
Boiled egg with wholemeal
toast and low-fat spread
Apple

Lunch
Baked potato with
Homemade Baked Beans
in Tomato Sauce (page 75)
Orange juice

Afternoon snack
2 Fruit and Nut Cookies
(page 131)
Kiwi fruit

Evening
Macaroni and Broccoli
Cheese (page 35)
Side salad

Sunday

Breakfast
Grilled lean back bacon
(or vegetarian sausage)
Grilled tomatoes
Wholemeal toast with
low-fat spread

Lunch
Lean roast beef
Roast potatoes (cooked
in groundnut oil)
Carrots and green beans
Plum Crumble (page 130)

Afternoon snack
Apple and orange segments

Evening
Homemade Baked Beans
(page 75) on toast

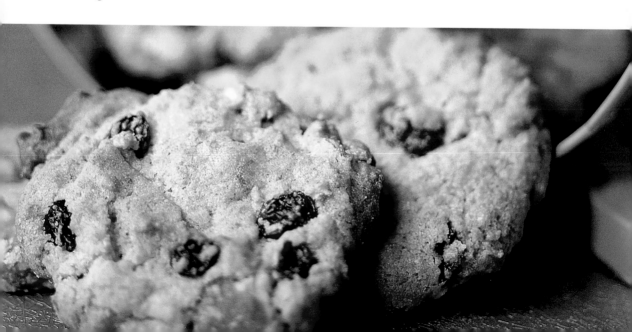

5 years+

Fruit and Nut Pasta Salad

Rich in nutrients, this easy salad is a good way to get children to eat nuts and seeds. It can also be made using couscous instead of pasta for a change.

100g dried wholewheat pasta shells
pinch of salt
1 red apple, cored and chopped
50g almonds
25g pine nuts
2 medium celery stalks, chopped
1 small red pepper, deseeded and chopped
50g red or white seedless grapes, halved
2 tbsp French dressing

1 Cook the pasta in lightly salted boiling water for 10 minutes, or until just tender, then drain. Tip into a bowl and allow to cool.
2 Add the chopped apple and all the other ingredients to the cooled pasta, stirring well to combine. Serve immediately or refrigerate for up to 24 hours.

2 servings

Good source of: protein, complex carbohydrates, essential fats, vitamins B1, B3, C, E, potassium, magnesium

Special diets: suitable for vegetarians including vegans, dairy-free

Not suitable for freezing

- 2 servings

- Good source of: protein, complex carbohydrates, vitamins B1, B3, potassium, magnesium, iron

- Special diets: suitable for vegetarians including vegans, dairy-free, wheat- and gluten-free, nut- and seed-free

- Not suitable for freezing

TIP
Cooked rice can be stored in a covered bowl in the fridge for up to 24 hours, but no longer.

Apricot and Brown Rice Salad

If properly cooked, brown basmati rice isn't at all tough and children enjoy its nutty flavour.

75g brown basmati rice
100g canned brown or green lentils, drained
5cm piece of cucumber, finely chopped
1 medium celery stalk, chopped
50g dried organic ready-to-eat apricots, chopped
2 tsp finely chopped fresh parsley
2 tbsp light olive oil
1 tbsp orange juice
pinch of salt
black pepper (optional)

1 Cook the rice in boiling water until tender, drain and leave to cool.
2 In a bowl, combine the rice with the lentils, cucumber, celery, apricots and parsley.
3 Whisk the olive oil, orange juice and seasoning together to make a dressing, drizzle over the salad and toss to mix. Serve immediately.

12 mths+

5 years+

Chicken and Pasta Salad

This salad is equally good warm or cold. It uses wholewheat pasta, which provides more fibre, B vitamins and minerals than plain pasta, but use the latter if you prefer. *(Illustrated on page 119)*

100g dried wholewheat penne pasta, or other shapes
pinch of salt
200g skinless chicken breast fillet
1 tbsp light olive oil
2 tbsp French dressing
1 small red onion, peeled and cut into 8 wedges
100g beef tomato, cut into 8 wedges
1 medium yellow pepper, deseeded and cut into 8 pieces
few fresh basil leaves (optional)

1 Cook the pasta in lightly salted boiling water until barely tender, about 10 minutes; drain and cool.
2 Meanwhile, heat the grill to medium-high. Cut the chicken into large bite-sized pieces and place in a bowl. Add the olive oil and toss to coat, then lay in the grill pan.
3 Add 1 tbsp French dressing to the oil left in the bowl. Add the onion, tomato and pepper, toss well, then spread amongst the chicken.
4 Grill for 10 minutes, or until the chicken and vegetables are golden, then turn everything and cook on the other side for 6–8 minutes, spooning over any juices. Check that the chicken is cooked right through: pierce with a knife tip – the juices should be clear, not at all pink, and the deepest piece of flesh must not still be pink.
5 Combine the chicken and vegetables with the pasta in a serving bowl. Drizzle over the pan juices, scatter over a few basil leaves if you like and serve warm or allow to cool.

2 servings

Good source of: protein, complex carbohydrates, carotenoids, vitamins B3, B6, E, potassium, selenium

Special diets: dairy-free, nut- and seed-free

Not suitable for freezing

- 4 servings
- Good source of: protein, carotenoids, vitamins A, B6, B12, folate, C, D, E, potassium, iodine
- Special diets: suitable for vegetarians, dairy-free, wheat- and gluten-free, nut- and seed-free
- Not suitable for freezing

5 years+

Baked Eggs and Peppers

This is an excellent lunch or supper dish, rich in vitamin C and very colourful. When cooked, the peppers become very sweet and I think this is why children really enjoy the taste. The dish isn't suitable for very young children as it contains partially cooked egg. Accompany with some good bread for a complete meal.

1½ tbsp light olive oil
4–6 mixed red, orange and yellow peppers, deseeded and thinly sliced
1 medium onion, thinly sliced
2 large ripe tomatoes, halved and sliced
1 tsp ground cumin
pinch of salt
black pepper
4 large best-quality eggs
drizzle of olive oil (basil-infused if possible)
few fresh basil leaves (optional)

1 Preheat the oven to 190°C/gas 5. Heat the olive oil in a non-stick frying pan and sauté the peppers and onion over a medium heat for about 5 minutes. Turn the heat down and cook, stirring from time to time, for a further 15 minutes, or until the vegetables are soft and lightly golden. Add the tomatoes, cumin and seasoning, stir to combine and cook for a further 5 minutes.

2 Spoon the mixture into 4 individual ovenproof dishes and make a well in the centre of each. Break an egg into each well and drizzle a little over the yolk of each one.

3 Cover with foil and bake for 12 minutes, or until the eggs are lightly set but the yolks are still runny. Scatter over a few basil leaves to serve if you like.

5 years+

Vegetable Burgers

These are a change from meat burgers. Don't be put off by the long list of ingredients – they are actually quick and easy to put together.

1½ tbsp light olive oil
1 medium (100g) onion, finely chopped
1 small carrot (50g), peeled and grated
1 garlic clove, peeled and finely chopped (optional)
1 small canned sweet red pepper, well drained and finely chopped
1 level tsp mixed dried herbs
1 level tsp season-all seasoning
1 level tsp ground cumin
2 tsp sun-dried tomato purée
dash of light soy sauce
200g canned chickpeas, well drained
50g ground almonds
2 tsp light tahini (sesame seed paste)
50g wholemeal breadcrumbs (approximately)

4 servings

Good source of: protein, complex carbohydrates, vitamins B2, B3, folate, E, potassium, calcium, magnesium

Special diets: suitable for vegetarians including vegans, dairy-free

Suitable for freezing

VARIATIONS

• Use mashed kidney beans or cannellini beans, or even cooked red lentils, instead of the chickpeas if you like, or a combination of these.

• For those who can't eat nuts, omit the ground almonds and make up the weight with extra chickpeas plus 2 tsp olive oil.

• For children who can't eat seeds, omit the tahini paste and add a little extra sun-dried tomato purée instead.

1 Heat half the oil in a non-stick frying pan and sauté the onion and carrot over a medium heat for 8 minutes, or until soft and translucent.
2 Add the garlic, if using, and the sweet pepper, and stir-fry for a minute or two, then add the herbs, seasoning, cumin, tomato purée and soy sauce, and combine well. Turn the heat off and set aside.
3 In a bowl, mash the chickpeas well, then add the ground almonds, tahini and the contents of the frying pan. Combine well and add enough breadcrumbs to make a firm mix. Form into 4 burgers.
4 Brush a griddle, grill or non-stick frying pan with the remaining oil and cook the burgers on a medium high heat for 2–3 minutes on each side, or until golden brown. (Or, bake on an oiled baking tray in an oven preheated to 200°C/gas 6 for 10 minutes, or until golden.)

About 4 servings

Good source of: protein, complex carbohydrates, vitamins A, B1, B3, B6, B12, folate, D, potassium, magnesium, iodine, selenium

Special diets: wheat- and gluten-free, nut- and seed-free

Not suitable for freezing

TIPS
• The finished kedgeree should be slightly moist, so if the rice seems too dry towards the end of cooking time, add a little more hot stock to the pan.
• For a gluten-free diet, if you use bought stock make sure it is gluten-free.

5 years+

Tuna and Egg Kedgeree

This kedgeree can also be made using white fish, e.g. cod or haddock, or smoked haddock, though smoked foods shouldn't be eaten often.

10g butter
2 tsp light olive oil
2 shallots, finely chopped
200g fresh tuna steak (or canned in water)
200g (dry weight) brown basmati rice
1 tsp korma or other mild curry powder (optional)
400ml vegetable stock (page 32) or good-quality fish stock
3 medium eggs
75g petit pois, defrosted
1 tbsp chopped fresh parsley

1 Heat the butter and olive oil together in a large non-stick frying pan (with a lid) and sauté the shallots over a medium heat for 6–8 minutes, or until softened. Push them to the sides of the pan.
2 Add the fresh tuna steak and cook for 1½ minutes on each side, then remove with a slotted spatula (leaving onion in pan); set aside.
3 Add the rice and curry powder, if using, to the pan, stir well, then add the stock and bring to a simmer. Turn the heat down, put the lid on and cook gently for about 20 minutes, or until almost cooked.
4 Meanwhile, boil the eggs for 8 minutes, rinse under cold water, shell and cut into quarters. Flake the tuna into bite-sized pieces.
5 When the rice is about 3 minutes from being cooked, add the peas and return the seared tuna to the rice pan (or add canned tuna). Stir in most of the parsley, then put the lid back on and cook for 3 minutes.
6 Serve topped with the hard-boiled egg quarters and garnished with the remaining parsley.

Chicken Enchiladas

For young primary school children with smaller appetites, use mini tortillas.

1 tbsp light olive oil
1 red onion, thinly sliced
1 red pepper, deseeded and thinly sliced
1 medium courgette, topped, tailed and thinly sliced
1 large garlic clove, peeled and well crushed
400g skinless chicken fillet, cut into thin slices
100g Cheddar cheese, grated
8 (40g) wheat tortillas
1 recipe-quantity Tomato Sauce (page 47)

1 Preheat the oven to 180°C/gas 4. Heat the olive oil in a non-stick frying pan and sauté the onion, pepper and courgette over a medium heat for about 10 minutes, or until everything is soft and turning golden, adding the garlic for the last 2 minutes.
2 Push the vegetables to the edges of the pan and add the chicken fillet. Sauté for 5 minutes, or until the chicken is golden and cooked through, then stir in half of the Cheddar cheese and mix everything together well.
3 Place one-eighth of the mixture on each tortilla and roll up, then place them side by side snugly in an ovenproof dish. Pour over the tomato sauce, sprinkle the remaining cheese over the top and bake for 20 minutes, or until the top is bubbling and the enchiladas are piping hot.

4 servings

Good source of: protein, carotenoids, vitamins B3, B6, C, E, potassium, calcium, selenium

Special diets: nut- and seed-free

Suitable for freezing, but best eaten fresh

- **4 servings**
- **Good source of: protein, vitamins B2, B3, B6, B12, potassium, iron, zinc**
- **Special diets: dairy-free, wheat- and gluten-free, nut- and seed-free**
- **Not suitable for freezing**

5 years+

Lamb and Cherry Tomato Kebabs

These simple kebabs are tasty and useful for children who are put off by large pieces of meat. They can be barbecued as well as grilled, or they can even be cooked in the oven. You'll need wooden kebab sticks – pre-soak these in cold water to prevent them scorching.

700g lean lamb fillet, cut into bite-sized cubes
1 tbsp light olive oil
juice of ½ lemon
1 level tsp dried rosemary
1 level tsp dried thyme
1 large garlic clove, peeled and well crushed
¼ tsp garam masala (optional)
pinch of salt
8 large cherry tomatoes
4 medium shallots, peeled and halved

1 Place the lamb in a shallow non-metallic dish. Mix together the olive oil, lemon juice, herbs, garlic, garam masala and salt, then pour over the lamb and mix to coat well. Leave to marinate for an hour or two if possible.

2 Heat the grill to medium-high. Remove the lamb from the marinade with a slotted spoon. Add the cherry tomatoes and shallot halves to the marinade and toss to coat.

3 Thread the lamb, shallots and tomatoes on to 4 wooden kebab sticks. Cook the kebabs for about 10 minutes, turning and basting with the marinade from time to time, until cooked through and evenly coloured.

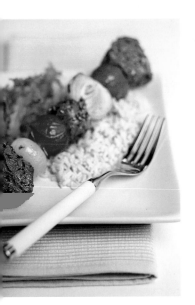

5 years+

Plum Crumble

A crumble is never going to be a low-calorie affair, but this one makes a nutritious pudding in winter.

800g ripe red plums, stoned and quartered
40g sugar
½ tsp ground cinnamon
125g wholemeal flour
50g butter or vegan margarine
40g soft brown sugar
40g chopped mixed nuts

1 Preheat the oven to 180°C/gas 4. Tip the plums into a baking dish and toss with the sugar and cinnamon. Sprinkle with 1 tbsp water.
2 Put the flour into a bowl and rub in the butter or margarine with your fingertips until it resembles breadcrumbs, then stir in the brown sugar and nuts and sprinkle this topping over the fruit.
3 Bake for 45 minutes, or until the crumble topping is golden and the juice begins to bubble up around the sides.

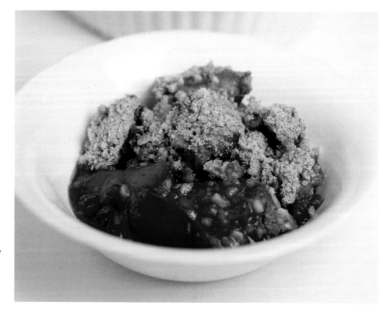

4–6 servings

Good source of: carotenoids, vitamins B1, B3, B6, E, potassium, magnesium, selenium

Special diets: suitable for vegetarians including vegans, dairy-free

Suitable for freezing, but best frozen before baking

Makes 30

Good source of: vitamins A, B1, B3, B6, B12, folate, D, E, magnesium, iron

Special diets: suitable for vegetarians, dairy-free

Not suitable for freezing

5 years+

Fruit and Nut Cookies

These are delicious after-school snacks. For children with a nut allergy, you can substitute 75g rolled oats for the peanut butter. For vegan children, use vegan margarine instead of the butter. *(Illustrated on page 121)*

cooking oil spray
125g vegetarian margarine
150g golden caster sugar
1 medium egg
75g wholemeal flour
75g plain white flour
½tsp baking powder
pinch of salt
125g crunchy peanut butter
100g sultanas
75g chopped dried ready-to-eat apricots

1 Preheat the oven to 190°C/gas 5 and spray two heavy-duty non-stick baking sheets with the oil.

2 In a bowl, combine the fat, sugar, egg, flours, baking powder, salt and peanut butter until well mixed, then stir in the sultanas and apricots. Spoon the mixture on to the baking sheets in 30 small spoonfuls, leaving enough room between them so they won't touch as they spread during cooking.

3 Bake for 15 minutes. Allow to cool a little, then place on wire racks to finish cooling. Store the cookies in an airtight tin.

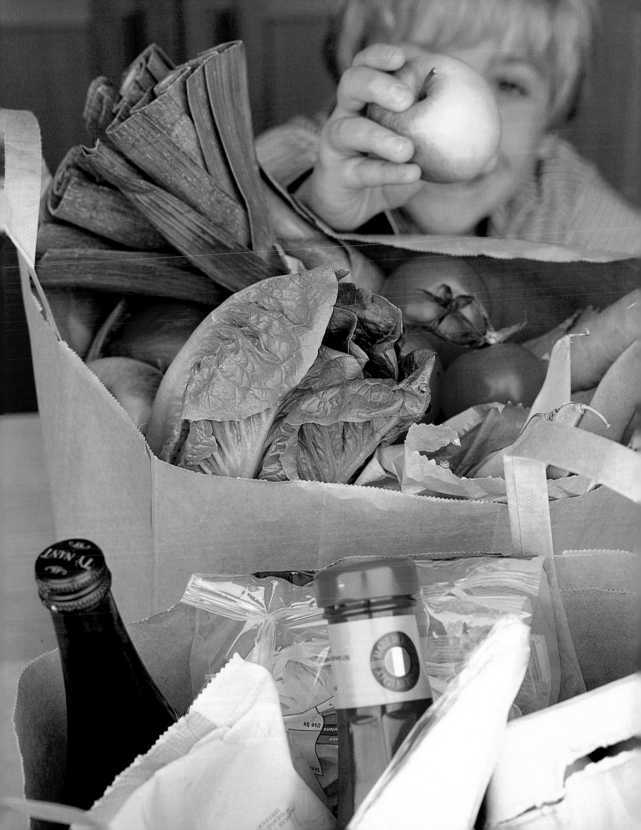

A–Z of child health & diet

In this section of the book you will find all of the information you need to know about particular topics related to your children's health and their diet. The subjects range from nutrients (e.g. vitamins and minerals) and types of foods (e.g. organic food) to health topics (e.g. eczema and food allergies) and well-being (e.g. fussy eating and food refusal).

For easy reference, I have presented the topics in alphabetical order. If there is any subject you want to know about, simply look here first. At the end of each entry, you will find references to related topics if applicable. If you have any significant concerns about your child's health, growth or development, then you should seek advice from your doctor.

ADDITIVES
see Food Additives

ADHD (Attention Deficit Hyperactivity Disorder)

Other names, and related names, for this disorder in children include hyperactivity, HKD (hyperkinetic disorder) and ADD (attention deficit disorder). To simplify matters, the umbrella term 'hyperactivity' is used here.

Hyperactivity is diagnosed, according to the Royal College of Physicians (RCP), as 'developmentally inappropriate levels' of inattention and difficulty in concentrating, excessive and/or disorganized levels of activity and impulsive behaviour. These symptoms should have persisted for at least 6 months, first start in children before the age of 6 or 7, must be present in more than one setting (e.g. at home and at school), must cause significant functional impairment and not be better accounted for by other disorders (e.g. depression or schizophrenia).

Prevalence of hyperactivity has been estimated by different bodies at between 1% and 17% of school age children in the UK. It is estimated that 1 in 20 children aged between 6 and 16 have ADHD. Boys are 4 times more likely to have hyperactivity than girls.

If you think your child may be hyperactive, you should take him or her to see your doctor. There is some evidence, however, that diet can play a role. Much attention is focused on the role of food additives. One study found that in some children certain food chemicals could cause reactions within 30 minutes. Another study of 3-year-olds found that significant changes in children's hyperactive behaviour could be produced by the removal of colourings and additives from their diet.

Children with hyperactivity have been found to be more thirsty than other children, and to have a higher incidence of eczema, asthma and other allergies.

The UK Hyperactive Children's Support Group recommends eliminating artificial food colourings, flavourings and preservatives and certain other foods – including a long list of fruits. However, the RCP says on current evidence it isn't possible to recommend diets that restrict or eliminate refined sugar and artificial additives for children with ADHD/HKD. Neither do they support the idea that supplementation with minerals such as zinc, iron or magnesium will help treat hyperactivity.

On the positive side, there is convincing evidence that supplementation with long-chain omega-3 essential fatty acids does help some children. This may be true particularly of those with low levels of the essential fats. Another theory is that the brain may have trouble converting essential polyunsaturated fats into the very-long-chain polyunsaturates, for instance DHA and EPA found in oily fish.

The UK Institute of Child Health says that modifying the diet might help, and that up to half of the children affected by hyperactivity can be helped by behavioural therapy alone.

See also: Behavioural Problems p139, Dyslexia and Dyspraxia p154, Food Additives p159, Contacts p219.

ALLERGIES
see Food Allergies

Anaemia

Anaemia is a lack of haemoglobin, which carries oxygen around the bloodstream. The major cause of anaemia in childhood is iron deficiency, which is usually due to too little of the mineral in the diet. Girls around puberty are more at risk of iron-deficiency anaemia.

The symptoms: A pale colour, tiredness, lethargy, headaches, dizziness and – when the anaemia is severe – a shortness of breath. If severe anaemia isn't treated, mental and physical developmental may be impaired.

What to do: If you think your child may be anaemic, take him or her to the doctor who will probably do a blood test. If lack of iron in the diet is the cause, the doctor may prescribe supplements and/or a diet high in iron-rich foods, such as red meat, dark leafy green vegetables, pulses, whole grains, dried fruits and seeds. Iron is better absorbed if eaten with a good source of vitamin C, e.g. citrus fruit or juice, or red peppers.

See also: Minerals for sources of iron p186, Vitamins for sources of vitamin C p216.

ANAPHYLACTIC SHOCK
see Food Allergies

Antioxidants

'Antioxidant' is a term used to describe a range of vitamins, minerals and plant chemicals, which 'mop up' free radicals within the body and thus help to prevent certain diseases and slow signs of ageing. Free radicals are particles produced in the body as a result of normal living. However, in certain circumstances – for example, when people are ill, under stress, smoke or take a great deal of physical activity, or when they get old – the production of free radicals increases and it is thought that a surfeit of free radicals is linked with increased risk of diseases, including cancers and coronary heart disease. The damaging effects of free radicals can be counteracted by antioxidants, which in effect neutralize them.

Healthy children are not at as great a risk from free radicals as are the ill or elderly, but nevertheless should be encouraged to eat foods rich in the antioxidant vitamins, minerals and plant compounds regularly as part of an overall healthy diet.

The most important antioxidants:
→ Vitamins: A, C, E and Beta-carotene
→ Minerals: Zinc and Selenium
→ Plant chemicals: the Flavonoid group

See also: Convalescence p149, Minerals p185, Phytochemicals p195, Vitamins p213.

Anxiety

Most children go through periods of feeling anxious or nervous and can suffer stress through life events such as moving home, breakdown of relationships within the family, or having friendship or school problems. If an anxious child has trouble sleeping, this will exacerbate the problem.

A diet rich in the vitamin B group, and the minerals calcium and magnesium is known to help the nervous system to cope – calcium has been called nature's tranquillizer. Prolonged stress depletes the body of the water-soluble B and C vitamins, so it's a good idea to make sure an anxious or stressed child has a diet rich in these. Short-term anxiety can be eased a little with a high-carbohydrate meal or snack, such as pasta, baked potato or a sandwich. Carbohydrate foods are known to have a soporific effect. Exercise also helps to calm the nerves by releasing endorphins.

A child who is stressed out may lose his or her appetite but it is counterproductive to try to force a child to eat at such times. Indeed, stress can sometimes induce feelings of nausea, exacerbating the problem.

Tips for feeding an anxious child
→ Offer very small portions of foods that are normally favourites.
→ Avoid anything too rich – chocolate cake, fatty meats, cheese sauce, etc.
→ Provide food in a relaxed atmosphere: music – even upbeat – can ease nerves. If eating as a family, keep the conversation light and chatty.
→ Provide a variety of different foods 'buffet-style' and let the child pick what they want.
→ Serve a meal after the child has taken exercise, outdoors if the weather permits.
→ Don't worry too much as appetite usually returns before long. However, if the child is stressed for more than a few days, you need to try to resolve the cause and seek your doctor's advice if necessary.

The family that eats together...
One Spanish study found that families who don't eat meals together are more likely to produce children with psychological problems than families who do.

See also: Appetite Loss (below), Fussy Eating and Food Refusal p174, Insomnia p180, Supplements p208.

Appetite loss
In the short term, almost all children, like adults, will go through periods of having a small or poor appetite. This can be because they are ill or perhaps because they are experiencing negative emotions – such as worry, fear and stress.

Eating less than is normal, or appropriate, for a few days – or even weeks – is no great cause for worry, especially if you know the cause. Try to deal with the cause and the appetite problems should resolve. Check that your child isn't filling up between meals on fatty or sugary foods or drinks, which would dull the appetite for mealtimes.

Long-term poor appetite – or 'restrictive eating' as it is sometimes described – is when a child eats smaller than average portions for her or his age, or may not want to eat as often as other children, or may refuse to eat at normal mealtimes. The result is that fewer calories than average will be consumed. This will usually result in the child being thinner than average and can, if severe, restrict growth and normal development. Poor appetite is quite common in pre-school and primary-school age children.

What to do? Take your child to see the doctor to ensure that he or she is healthy and a suitable weight. If this is the case then nothing more needs to be done. Trying to force, persuade or encourage the child to eat bigger portions – or to eat more frequently – makes no difference, and may make matters worse. Simply attempt, without any comment or discussion, to provide your child with foods that offer a high level of vitamins, minerals and protein, even in small portions, rather than letting the child fill up on sweets, fizzy drinks or crisps. This will help ensure he or she meets the recommended levels of nutrients.

If the doctor feels that the child's growth is being restricted or health impaired, then he or she will discuss the options with you. The good news is that, in the long term, poor eaters do usually find their appetite improves. They may stay slim and become slim adults, but this needn't be linked to poor health.

See also: Feeding Problems p55, Convalescence p149, Fussy Eating and Food Refusal p174, Illness, feeding during p180, Underweight p210.

Apples

Compared with many other fruits, apples are a good but not excellent source of vitamin C, the content of which can vary considerably, depending on how long the apples have been in storage before being bought, and on storage at home.

Apples have been found to help lower blood cholesterol and improve lung function, probably due to their high content of the phytochemical quercetin, and of another plant compound, catechin, both of which are members of the flavonoid group.

Apples contain the mineral boron, which helps to prevent calcium loss and may help to build good bone structure.

See also: Asthma (below), Fruit p173, Phytochemicals p195, Vitamins p213.

Asthma

Asthma is a disease of the airways that carry air into and out from the lungs. These tubes become sensitive and inflamed and, when an asthma attack is triggered, the airways swell making it hard to breathe. In severe cases asthma can be life-threatening.

Rates of asthma have doubled in this country in the past 10 years and now about 1 in 5 children are affected, making it the most common long-term childhood illness. The causes are varied, but diet seems to play a significant role. Indeed, some experts believe that diet is the biggest factor contributing to increased asthma in wealthier countries, where there is a move away from natural towards fast foods.

Studies indicate that a diet rich in fruit, vegetables and perhaps oily fish, which tends to be anti-inflammatory, can help prevent or minimize the condition. The National Asthma Campaign (NAC) advises that regular intake of fresh fruit can protect against asthma and other lung diseases. Omega-3 fish oil is known to have anti-inflammatory properties which may ease asthmatic symptoms, and there is evidence that low magnesium intake is associated with higher prevalence of asthma.

There is less research linking particular foods with increased risk of asthma, but studies have found that it could be linked to a high intake of omega-6 fats found in many vegetable and seed oils (e.g. corn, sunflower and safflower) and trans fats present in commercially manufactured foods. Omega-6 oils tend to be pro-inflammatory. However, this doesn't appear to apply to the very-long-chain omega-6s (highly unsaturated fatty acids), which may actually be beneficial.

For women planning a new pregnancy, taking antibiotics in pregnancy may increase the risk of the child developing asthma, as may smoking and a shortfall of vitamins C and E, while intake of oily fish and fish oils, rapeseed oil and soya bean oil have been linked with a reduction of wheezing in babies. Breast-feeding certainly seems to have a significant protective effect against the development of asthma.

The NAC says that food and drink are not common triggers for people with asthma, although food allergies can produce symptoms which can resemble an asthma attack. Some of the most common foods to produce such a reaction are dairy produce, shellfish, products containing food additives called sulphites (E numbers 220-227) and tartrazine (E102), and wheat, but a variety of other foods may cause asthmatic symptoms in susceptible individuals.

See also: Eczema p155, Essential Fatty Acids p156, Fats and Oils p157, Food Allergies p162, Obesity p189.

Autism

Research has found that two-thirds of autistic children have a deficiency in the omega-3 fatty acids, and those who were fed fish oils made significant improvement – for example, in their concentration and sleep patterns. It was also found that children with Asperger's syndrome, a condition related to autism, had low blood levels of omega-3s.

See also: Behavioural Problems p139, Essential Fatty Acids p156, Fish p159.

Bananas

Bananas are one of the best sources of potassium, which helps to regulate body fluids. They also contain a type of dietary fibre known as fructo-oligosaccharides (FOS). This helps to promote healthy bacteria in the gut and may be useful for children who have frequent stomach upsets and constipation. Bananas are easily digested and popular with most children. They are one of the few fruits with a good starch content, allowing for a slow release of energy – the carbohydrate in most fruits is mainly in the form of fruit sugars.

See also: Carbohydrates p144, Constipation p148, Dietary Fibre p152, Fruit p173.

BEANS, DRIED
see Pulses

Bedwetting

Bedwetting, or enuresis, is a common problem in young children and can persist well into the primary school years. Dietary factors are rarely the main cause but if your child is prone, it is obviously worth managing their levels of hydration by providing plenty to drink during the day rather than giving a lot to drink in the hour or two before bedtime. A carbohydrate-rich snack at bedtime may also help prevent bedwetting, as the carbohydrate, such as bread or a scone, literally 'mops up' liquid and diminishes the need to go to the toilet. Avoid natural diuretic foods in the evening – these include celery, melon, asparagus, citrus fruits and watercress.

Some research indicates that bedwetting is more common in obese children.

If your child begins to wet the bed after having been dry, and especially if he or she begins to drink a lot more than previously, take him or her to the doctor, who should consider doing a test for diabetes.

See also: Carbohydrates p144, Diabetes p151, Obesity p189.

Behavioural problems

Can diet influence children's mood and behaviour? ADHD, depression, dyslexia and dyspraxia, nerves and anxiety are all covered elsewhere in this A–Z section. But several other, or related, behavioural problems, such as mood swings, irritability and even delinquency, have been linked with diet.

Food additives

There is some research to indicate that food colourings (E numbers and others) and, to a lesser extent, other additives, such as preservatives and flavourings, may cause behavioural changes or problems in children.

(Further information can be found in the ADHD and Food Additives entries.) One large primary school in the UK banned additives in school meals. Consequently the children behaved better at school and slept better at night according to their parents. However, as yet, there is only slight scientific evidence for a link between behaviour and additives. **My advice?** Because many of the additive-rich foods and drinks are also those low in nutritional value, a diet which limits these items makes sense.

Sugar

Many believe that there is a link between intake of sugar and sugary foods and behaviour disruption, though this is widely disputed. There is some scientific rationale behind the sugar/bad behaviour theory. If a child eats a diet high in sugar, this may cause blood glucose levels to rise quickly, giving a 'high', which can make a child excitable. Then, as insulin is released, the levels may plummet and the child may feel unusually drowsy and perhaps unable to concentrate. Then, to stop the levels falling further, adrenaline may be released in the body, which can increase irritability. This pattern depends on what else the child has eaten, etc., but in theory 'sugar overload' behaviour is possible.

My advice? Again, as sugar is a nutrient-poor food, limiting its use won't cause any problems in your child's diet and so it is worth a try. If you do offer sugary foods or drinks, let your child have them as part of a nutritious meal to limit any side-effects by keeping blood sugar levels more even.

It is also worth pointing out that although the brain needs sugar (glucose) to function properly, the body converts foods into sugar as necessary; actual sugar isn't required for blood glucose to be made.

Nutrition and delinquency

An interesting study of school children found that those with higher levels of the long-chain omega-3s, DHA and EPA, in their bodies had lower scores for both violent aggressive behaviour and anger. This same study found that very-long-chain omega-6 acid actually increased anger and aggression. So it seems that it is the omega-3 fatty acids which effect positive changes in behaviour and other problems such as ADHD, rather than the omega-6s.

These studies reinforce the notion that a good well-balanced diet is important for proper brain functioning, which is, of course, where 'behaviour' begins. If, on the other hand, your child's diet contains an optimum amount of vitamins, minerals and fatty acids, it is unlikely that giving him or her even more will effect any further improvement.

Dehydration

Children sometimes don't drink enough hydrating fluids, especially when they are at school, and this can result in lethargy, lack of concentration and irritability. Try to ensure that your child's school has a facility for drinking water available all the time and when children are out and about, encourage them to take a bottled water drink with them.

Eating as a family

There is evidence to suggest that children from families who rarely eat meals together suffer from more psychological problems than those who do. Try to eat as a family, as often as you can, and make mealtimes enjoyable and relaxed.

Exercise

Exercise may be as important as diet in improving children's behaviour. A recent experiment found that with at least half an hour a day of sports, primary school children were quicker to settle down in class, more enthusiastic and less disruptive.

See also: The School Day p110, ADHD p134, Brain Power p141, Drinks p153, Dyslexia and Dyspraxia p154, Essential Fatty Acids p156, Fats and Oils p157, Food Additives p159, Food Allergies p162, Sugar and Sweeteners p205.

Berry fruits

All berry fruits are low in calories and have a good vitamin C content. Most are a good source of dietary fibre and are high in natural sugars. Most are also a good source of ellagic acid, which is both anti-cancer and a strong antioxidant. Blueberries (1st), blackberries (2nd) and strawberries (5th) are ranked in the 'top five' for antioxidant activity in foods. Raspberries are a good source of folate.

Most children enjoy berries. Try serving them with Greek yoghurt or natural fromage frais, which are lower in fat than whipped or double cream, or blend them into drinks such as smoothies, or purée and stir into natural yoghurt for a healthy dessert.

See also: Antioxidants p135, Drinks recipes p102–3.

Bone health

Bones continue to grow and develop their density and strength until around the age of 30, after which bone density slowly begins to decline. About 45% of bone mass is built up in adolescence, and by the late teens the bones usually stop growing in length, thus deciding your child's final height.

A good bone structure helps minimize symptoms of osteoporosis in later life and reduces the risk of fractures. Although regular weight-bearing exercise (e.g. running around) is important to maximize bone density, diet is a major factor in bone development.

Bone consists of collagen plus minerals, mostly calcium and phosphate. Calcium is a major component of bone and a growing child's diet needs to be adequate in calcium-rich foods, such as dairy produce and dark leafy green vegetables.

Calcium helpers

Dietary calcium is not always well-absorbed by the body – 70% or more of it may be excreted in urine. As well as ensuring adequate intake, it is therefore important to help absorption as much as possible.

Vitamin D is needed to help calcium absorption and a deficiency of this vitamin can cause rickets. Calcium works with magnesium to form bone, so an adequate magnesium intake is also needed.

Essential fatty acids, such as fish and plant oils – are thought to play a role in calcium metabolism, and absorption of calcium from leafy green vegetables also seems to be better than that from dairy produce. A diet generally high in fruit and vegetables seems to favour calcium retention. Research has found a link between optimum vitamin E intake and bone density, while zinc is another important mineral to help build bone.

Calcium robbers

Similarly, certain foods and drinks decrease mineral absorption or increase excretion. A diet high in protein, especially animal protein, can increase calcium excretion. Caffeine, found mainly in coffee, cola drinks and tea, seems to cause small but significant increases in calcium excretion. And a diet high in salt increases the excretion of calcium in urine.

Perhaps the crucial factor for children is that a diet high in phosphates appears to limit calcium absorption. Carbonated drinks, soft drinks and processed foods can all contain high levels of phosphates. If your child has any kind of restrictive or special diet (e.g. vegan), it is very important that you ensure adequate intake of the nutrients vital for bone-building.

See also: Drinks p153, Minerals p185, Processed Foods p199.

Brain power

There has been much research to indicate that children's diet has a great influence over their brain power. A variety of trials have indicated that children who eat an optimum range of nutrients show improved IQ, concentration and memory. Most trials have focused on multi-nutrients, but some have suggested that specific vitamins and minerals seem particularly important, including vitamin C, iron and vitamin B12.

Is fish really brain food?

One important area of research is in the link between intelligence and very-long-chain fatty acids. Most research has focused on the omega-3 oils, DHA and EPA, which are provided by oily fish in the diet, and can also be made from the long-chain omega-3 fatty acid alpha-linolenic acid. DHA and other long-chain fats make up about 60% of the brain's material, so it is not really surprising that from the baby in the womb through to adulthood, a diet that contains plenty of these essential fats appears to boost brain power. Because our consumption of fish, especially oily fish, has decreased significantly it seems that these very-long-chain essential fats are often missing in our children's diets.

Other factors

There is some evidence that food additives may have an adverse effect on children's ability to concentrate. Caffeine-containing fizzy drinks have also been linked with poor concentration at school, since a diet high in caffeine causes children to sleep less well at night and become sleepy during the day.

A lack of water or other hydrating fluids can also induce lethargy and lack of concentration, so aim to ensure school children take plenty of water to drink during the day – one small bottle is not sufficient, especially in hot weather. Regular exercise has also been shown to boost brain function, enhancing mood, concentration and memory.

Blood sugar levels

There is plenty of evidence to show that children's academic work improves when they have regular nutritious meals. Those children who skip meals or who aren't given a good breakfast may have low blood sugar levels, which has a knock-on effect on the brain, as it uses blood sugars as its source of energy. All types of thinking use up the brain's energy supplies more quickly than was previously realized.

A significant proportion of school children never have a breakfast, yet this meal can improve educational performance, memory, concentration and problem-solving abilities. It is particularly important because of the long time-gap since the last meal.

See also: ADHD p134, Behavioural Problems p139, Drinks p153, Dyslexia and Dyspraxia p154, Essential Fatty Acids p156, Fats and Oils p157, Fish p159, Food Additives p159, Vitamins p213.

Bread

Bread is the major source of starchy carbohydrates in the Western diet and most is made from wheat grain. White bread contains up to 80% of the whole wheat grain but no outer layer (bran) or seed (germ). Because of this, it contains less fibre than wholegrain bread, and would contain less vitamins and minerals if it were not for the fact that in this country B vitamins, calcium and iron are added to the refined white flour to give it a better nutritional profile. The iron content of white bread, though, is still lower than that for wholemeal bread.

White, wholegrain and brown breads (which contain 85–90% of the whole grain) are nutritious foods for children, as are the range of breads made from flours other than wheat – e.g. dark or light rye breads, corn bread and so on. Most breads are low in fat, although enriched breads like croissants and garlic bread are not.

Most bread contains moderately high amounts of sodium, as it tends to taste very bland unless a reasonable amount of salt is added. This will only be a problem if your child has a lot of other high-salt foods in his or her diet.

Mass-produced bread usually contains more additives than you might imagine – bleaching agents, preservatives, GM-soya bean flour, and colourings such as caramel. To avoid these you will need to buy organic or traditional loaves.

A small proportion of children are allergic to, or intolerant of, one or more of the constituents of bread. Children who are allergic to the gluten in wheat, rye, barley or oats need to follow a special gluten-free diet. Other children may be intolerant of the yeast in bread and need to be given yeast-free bread. Soda bread is free from yeast, as are some – but not all – flatbreads. A few children are intolerant of wheat but not rye, barley or other grains. This is not the same as a gluten allergy. If you think your child may have an allergy or intolerance, see your doctor.

See also: Carbohydrates p144, Coeliac Disease p147, Food Allergies p162, Grains p175.

Cancer prevention

Bacup (www.cancerbacup.org.uk), the UK's leading cancer information service, has general guidelines on the type of healthy diet which may help to prevent some forms of cancer. These can be summarized as keeping to a reasonable body weight, eating less fat, sugar and salt, and eating vegetables, fruit and grains. The advice and eating plans in the first part of this book give basic healthy diets for children similar to these guidelines (with differences appropriate to different ages).

There has been little research specifically on childhood cancer and diet, but a prudent diet in childhood may improve your child's chances of avoiding cancer later in life. There are certainly indications that the higher the fruit consumption during childhood, the less likely the risk of developing cancer as an adult. A research study for the World Health Organization reported that 10% of all cancer cases in the developed world could be the result of people not eating enough fruit and vegetables. The clearest evidence of a link, they say, is for stomach and lung cancers.

As a significant number of children eat less than the recommended amounts of fruits and vegetables, encouraging your child to eat more is a positive way of helping them to good long-term health.

Canned foods

Although convenient, many canned foods have a poor nutritional profile, including ready-meals and processed meats. However, some are a nutritionally sound addition to the storecupboard, including the following:

→ **Canned pulses:** These are ideal for quick meals – especially when you forgot to soak the dried versions. Buy red kidney beans, black eye beans, cannellini beans, butter beans, chickpeas and lentils canned in water rather than brine. Nutritionally, they are similar to reconstituted dried pulses. Baked beans in tomato sauce are popular with children and they are a good source of protein, fibre, iron and magnesium. Standard baked beans are, however, high in salt and sugar, so opt for reduced sugar/salt versions.

→ **Canned fruits and vegetables:** These will have lost some of their vitamin C and B group content, but are useful as occasional standbys. Buy vegetables canned in water rather than brine (high in salt) and fruit canned in juice rather than syrup (high in sugar).

→ **Canned rice pudding and custard:** Use these as standbys for desserts. For many children it is better to opt for the low-fat versions. Serve with fruit for a balanced dessert.

→ **Pulse and/or vegetable soups:** Useful for an occasional fast lunch or snack, but note that many canned soups are too high in sodium (salt) to make a regular part of a child's diet.

→ **Canned whole or chopped tomatoes:** These are a storecupboard must, and they are rich in the antioxidant lycopene. Canned carrots are rich in the antioxidant beta-carotene, which is better absorbed in canned or cooked carrots than in raw ones.

See also: Antioxidants p135, Processed Foods p199, Salt p203.

Carbohydrates

Carbohydrate is one of the 'macronutrients' (major nutrients), along with fat and protein. This means that it supplies energy (in the form of kilocalories, commonly known as calories) in the diet, at 3.75 calories per gram of carbohydrate. Indeed, carbohydrates are the main source of energy for most people, including children, at around 50% of the total calorie content of the diet.

There are two main types of carbohydrate – starches and sugars. Of total carbohydrates, starch contributed 55% of intake and sugars the remainder.

For good health, much of a child's carbohydrate intake should be in the form of starches rather than too much sugar – especially what is sometimes known as 'non-milk extrinsic sugars' – i.e. those added to food in cooking or preparation, or at table. Currently, children in this country eat too much of this extrinsic sugar. The other categories of sugars in the diet are 'intrinsic sugars' – i.e. those found as a natural part of the plant, e.g. in fruits – and milk sugars, found as a natural element of milk.

The main source of starches in a child's diet are grain foods like bread, cereals, pasta, rice and couscous, root vegetables such as potatoes, and pulses like kidney beans and baked beans. Most fruits don't contain starch, the exception being bananas, while most vegetables contain small or moderate amounts of starch.

The natural starchy plant-based foods are sometimes called 'complex carbohydrates'.

Refining these carbs – as in white bread, white rice and plain pasta – removes some of the fibre and nutrients from the plant and may alter its Glycaemic Index and its effect upon the blood sugars. However, these refined foods are still an important part of most children's diets and may even be more suitable than unrefined starches for some – the very young children, children with a poor appetite and/or those who are underweight.

The simplest way to ensure that your child eats plenty of starchy carbohydrates without too much added fat or sugar, is to restrict the intake of cakes, biscuits, pies and pastries, fried foods such as chips and crisps, and sugary and/or fatty breakfast cereals.

See also: Bread p142, Dietary Fibre p152, Grains p175, Obesity p189 for information on the Glycaemic Index, Potatoes p198, Sugar and Sweeteners p205.

Carrots

Carrots are one of the richest sources of the carotenoid group of plant compounds in the diet. These antioxidants have been linked with improved lung function and the health of the eyes, skin and immune system. Diets that include plenty of carotenoid-rich vegetables have been linked to a reduced risk of some cancers in adults.

The body's absorption of the beta-carotene content is improved if the carrots are cooked, and also when eaten with a little fat, so serve carrots with a dash of olive oil or a small knob of butter, or with a little oily dressing in a salad or as part of a stir-fry.

See also: Phytochemicals p195, Vegetables p212.

Cheese

Most types of cheese are an important source of calcium for bone development and health in children and, to a lesser extent, protein, as well as some B vitamins and vitamin A, but they can also be high in fat, saturated fat and salt. Cheese aimed at children – like triangles of soft cheese spread and cheese slices – tend to be very high in sodium.

In general, full-fat hard cheeses, such as Cheddar, are high in fat and sodium, but also high in calcium and protein, while full-fat soft cheeses, such as cream cheese, are high in fat but contain less calcium and protein. Low-fat soft cheeses contain reasonable amounts of protein, but are low in calcium and vitamins compared with hard cheeses.

Cheese doesn't contain any starch; its carbohydrate content is all in the form of milk sugars. When serving cheese to children, you need to weigh its positives (calcium, protein, vitamins) against its fat and sodium (salt) content. At least some of the time, try to choose the medium-fat cheeses such as Brie, mozzarella and feta, which contain good amounts of calcium and protein without too much of the fat.

For vegetarian children, you need to choose cheese without rennet in it – these days there is a wide range of rennet-free cheeses, both hard and soft, which will be labelled as such. For children with an intolerance to cows' milk, there are several cheeses available made from ewes' or goats' milk. Hard cheese, which contains an enzyme called tyramine, seems to cause migraine in some children – if this is the case, the soft cheeses, which don't contain tyramine, may not have this effect.

Avoid giving any cheese to babies under 6 months old. Soft mould-ripened cheese, such as Brie and Camembert, and blue cheeses should not be given to infants under 12 months old.

See also: Fats and Oils p157, Salt p203.

CHICKEN
see Poultry

Cholesterol

Although blood cholesterol levels have for a long time appeared to be an adult concern, in recent years Western children are increasingly showing signs of high cholesterol and early heart disease.

Cholesterol is mostly made in the liver and is transported in the blood by two proteins – low-density lipoprotein (LDL) and high-density lipoprotein (HDL). LDL cholesterol is known as 'bad' cholesterol because it can be deposited on the blood vessel walls, forming 'plaques', which may lead to narrowing of the arteries, increasing the risk of strokes, heart attacks and cardiovascular disease. HDL is known as the 'good' cholesterol because it actually helps to transport excess LDL cholesterol back to the liver.

A high intake of saturated and trans fats is thought to be more of a risk factor for high LDL cholesterol levels and heart disease than is actual cholesterol in the diet, although people diagnosed with high LDL levels and/or other risk factors for heart disease are usually advised to follow a low-cholesterol diet. High-cholesterol foods include liver and other offal foods, eggs, fatty meat, dairy produce and shellfish, and manufactured foods that include these items.

Children in this country eat more saturated and trans fats and have higher cholesterol levels than those in many other countries. Following a healthy balanced diet – low in saturated and trans fats and high in fruit and vegetables – from a young age can significantly reduce their risk of heart and circulatory problems later in life.

This is particularly important for a child with a parent who has high blood cholesterol levels and/or has had heart or circulatory disease. A simple blood cholesterol test carried out through your doctor can easily reveal whether or not the child has raised LDL levels.

A healthy cholesterol profile
The following factors can help to maintain a healthy blood cholesterol profile and reduce the risk of heart disease:
→ avoiding obesity and taking regular aerobic exercise.
→ eating a diet high in soluble fibre, including plenty of soya beans and other pulses.
→ eating sufficient omega-3 oils.
→ eating sufficient antioxidants (found mainly in fruits and vegetables).

See also: Dietary Fibre p152, Essential Fatty Acids p156, Fats and Oils p157, Heart Health p178.

Citrus fruits

Fresh citrus fruits are all good sources of vitamin C and phytochemicals, particularly flavonones, which are powerful antioxidants that have been shown to protect against heart disease, lung disease and some cancers.

Grapefruit contains different flavonones from oranges, which give it its characteristic bitter taste and have similar health-protecting properties. Lemons contain limonone, a phytochemical which, again, can help protect against heart disease and cancer. Oranges and lemons are good sources of pectin, a soluble fibre with a cholesterol-lowering effect.

You get more of the vital plant chemicals if you eat the fruit, including the pith, rather than just the juice. If giving freshly made citrus juices to your children, it's better to use a blender and make a smoothie, rather than a juice extractor that removes all the solids.

See also: Drinks p153, Fruit p173, Phytochemicals p195.

Coeliac disease

This disease is an inflammatory condition of the digestive system, which is caused by an inability to tolerate gluten, the protein found in wheat and rye grains, and similar proteins in barley and oats. Exposure to gluten damages the lining of the small intestine and this prevents the absorption of nutrients. Children who have coeliac disease may have weight loss or failure to grow, and there are usually other symptoms, such as diarrhoea, bloating and vomiting. The lack of absorption of iron can lead to anaemia and impaired calcium absorption can cause osteoporosis.

It seems that coeliac disease is often hereditary. First symptoms usually appear whenever grains containing gluten are introduced into the diet. However, symptoms may appear at any age and sometimes coeliac disease can go unnoticed for years.

The only 'cure' at the moment is to avoid gluten-containing products for the rest of the sufferer's life. The intestines will gradually repair themselves, the symptoms will disappear and health and growth should return to normal. If you suspect your child may have coeliac disease, take him or her to see your doctor, who will get proper tests carried out and refer you for further advice.

Avoiding gluten-containing foods is not easy, because gluten is present in many manufactured foods as well as the obvious ones, such as bread, cereals, cakes, biscuits and pasta. It is best to join a coeliac or gluten intolerance society, which is likely to produce an up-to-date list of gluten-free foods.

See also: Anaemia p135, Contacts p219.

Colds and coughs

Childhood colds and coughs are very common and normal, but their frequency, severity and/or duration may be influenced through diet. Colds, coughs and flu are caused by a viral infection and the infection is usually caught through contact with someone who already has it. It is hard to avoid this, but it is easier for a child to catch infections if his or her immune system is weakened.

The immune system can be strengthened, at least partially, by means of the right diet:
→ Include in the diet plenty of foods rich in Vitamin C – fresh fruit, salads and vegetables, and fruit juices. A low-dose supplement (250mg/day with bioflavonoids) at the first sign of a cold may help minimize symptoms and should be stopped once the cold is over.
→ Include plenty of zinc-rich foods in the diet – e.g. lean red meat, nuts, seeds, wheatgerm, Quorn, shellfish. You can buy vitamin C supplements that include zinc in the formula.
→ For older children who like aromatic flavours, ginger and garlic are said to help fight off infection and act as decongestants.
→ Persuade your child to drink plenty of fluids, such as water, diluted juices and hot water with honey and lemon. Honey is an antiseptic and can also be used on bread or in desserts and with fruit.

See also: Convalescence p149, Illness, feeding during p180.

Colic

Colic is a fairly common disorder in babies and is characterized by a great deal of crying and distress, caused by abdominal cramps and discomfort. This often occurs at a similar time each day, often in the early evening, and some experts say that it is more frequent in bottle-fed babies. Most cases of colic are over by the time the baby is 4–5 months old.

There is no definitive cause of colic that we yet know, although it is possible that, in some babies at least, it may be due to intolerance of one or more foods in the mother's diet (if she is breast-feeding) – e.g. cows' milk, wheat, nuts, eggs or seafood. It may also be caused by normal baby formula milk. If you suspect that your baby's colic is due to cows'-milk formula, see your doctor. He should refer you to a dietitian, who may change the baby to a different type of formula (e.g. soya formula).

Research has also shown that the type of fruit juice a mother gives her baby may affect colic. In a study of 'colicky' babies aged between 4 and 6 months, apple juice was found to be most difficult to digest, while white grape juice was one of the most well tolerated. This could be down to sorbitol, a natural non-absorbable sugar alcohol, present in apple juice but not grape juice.

Some parents have reported improvement in colic symptoms if the baby is given the herb fennel (available as a drink at chemists).

The Institute of Child Health recommends that breast-feeding mothers of colicky babies avoid citrus fruits and very sweet fruits, which may cause diarrhoea in the baby and exacerbate the stomach problems. For more information about colic and coping with it by non-dietary means, see your doctor.

Constipation

This is a common problem in childhood, and occurs when stools are dry and hard and can't be passed without difficulty. Once a child has been constipated this may set up a 'vicious circle', because he or she is reluctant to go to the toilet because of the discomfort.

It is wise to check with your doctor that the child's constipation isn't caused by any medical complaint. If the answer is 'no', a suitable diet high in soluble and insoluble fibre and fluids should almost certainly be able to cure the problem, although in the short term laxatives suitable for a child may be needed to get everything going again.

Measures to help relieve constipation:
→ At least 5 portions of fruit and veg a day. Prunes are well known for their laxative effect – they contain a compound called isatin, as well as sorbitol, another laxative. Other fruits high in sorbitol include plums, pears, cherries and apples. Rhubarb is another natural laxative and citrus fruits – especially oranges – seem to be too. Pulses and dried fruits are very high in total fibre and soluble fibre.
→ Provide wholegrain cereal products rather than refined (white). Brown rice, wholemeal bread and wholegrain pasta contain more fibre than refined versions.
→ At least 8 glasses of water a day, evenly spaced out. The fibre can't bulk and soften the stools without enough fluid.
→ Rose-hip syrup, olive oil and black strap molasses can all be given in a daily dose while the child has constipation.
→ Regular exercise. Exercise helps to stimulate the digestive system and bowels – many children don't get enough exercise. In the long term, it is unwise to simply keep on giving your child laxatives, as the bowels can come to rely on these.

See also: Dietary Fibre p152, Fruit p173, Vegetables p212.

Convalescence

When a child who has been ill is returning to normal health their appetite may return in full force, which is the body's way of making sure energy and nutrients are replaced. If this is the case, offer slightly bigger portions than normal and give plenty of healthy between-meal snacks, such as bananas, milk drinks, nuts and seeds (if older), and milk puddings.

If, however, during convalescence the appetite hasn't returned to normal, feed small portions as often as possible, opting for foods that most appeal to your child and that are easy to eat and digest (see below).

Offer vitamin-C rich fruits between meals, such as berry and citrus fruits. If the child has been on antibiotics, feed plenty of foods rich in oligosaccharides (found in soluble fibre), such as onions or Jerusalem artichokes. These act as prebiotics, stimulating the growth of healthy bacteria in the digestive system; tablets that do this are also available.

Foods for a recovering child:
→ Scrambled egg on wholemeal toast with chopped tomato mixed in.
→ Mashed potato with a poached egg on top, plus a glass of orange juice.
→ A homemade chicken or vegetable soup (recipes on pages 32, 68–70) with white bread.
→ Spaghetti in tomato sauce, grated cheese melted in.
→ Banana sandwich.
→ Good-quality cream of tomato soup from the chilled counter, served with a soft roll.
→ Macaroni cheese with sliced tomato on top.

→ Baked potato with grated cheese and butter.
→ Pasta tuna bake.
→ Hot milk with oatcake biscuits.

Perhaps the most important thing is to find out what your child feels he or she would like to eat, and work round that. Preparing a highly nutritious meal that the child won't eat will have you both feeling bad.

Make sure your child always has a drink of water by the bed. Once children are feeling better, they soon make up any lost weight and regain energy.

CONVENIENCE FOODS

see Processed Food, Ready Meals

CREAM

see Dairy Produce

Dairy alternatives

For vegan children or those who are allergic to dairy produce, soya milk, yoghurt and ice cream make good alternatives. Soya is a good low-fat source of protein but soya 'dairy' produce contains little calcium, unless labelled as 'calcium-enriched'. Some children who are allergic to cows' milk are able to tolerate goats' milk. Unweaned babies who can't tolerate cows'-milk formula and are not being breast fed may be given soya milk formula – this should be discussed with your doctor or midwife.

See also: The Vegetarian Infant p13, The Vegan Child p108, Milk p184, Yoghurt and Fromage Frais p218.

Dairy produce

Dairy produce – cows' milk, cream, yoghurt and cheese – varies in its nutritional profile according to the product and how it is made. Milk, yoghurt and hard cheese are good sources of calcium and protein, but hard cheeses are high in fat and saturated fat, and whole milk is also fairly high in fat. Cream cheeses and cream are very high in fat, and low in protein and calcium. Low-fat cheeses, like cottage cheese and fromage frais, are good sources of protein but quite low in calcium. Hard and blue cheeses are high in sodium.

Children under 5 need higher levels of fat in the diet than older children and adults, and they can be given full-fat dairy produce. Older children can be offered more moderate-fat dairy produce, such as semi-skimmed milk and mozzarella and Brie cheeses.

If you are watching your child's calorie, fat and saturated fat intake, limit cream and use lower-fat alternatives such as Greek yoghurt and 8%-fat fromage frais. Greek yoghurt is better in cooking, as fromage frais tends to curdle. For children who are overweight, skimmed milk, low-fat yoghurt and low-fat fromage frais can be used much of the time, with a little high-calcium full-fat cheese, such as Cheddar, to increase the calcium intake.

Most dairy produce is a good source of fat-soluble vitamin A and some B vitamins, but vitamin A is lost in the low-fat varieties. Children who don't eat dairy produce can substitute soya products and should ensure they get enough calcium in the diet.

See also: Cheese p145, Milk p184, Yoghurt, Fromage Frais p218.

Dehydration

Many children don't drink enough fluids to ensure that they are properly hydrated. Active children can easily become dehydrated, especially in hot weather or when doing sports or other aerobic exercise. They tend to get dehydrated more quickly than adults as they are smaller, sweat less and often don't pay attention to feelings of thirst.

Signs of dehydration include:
→ dark yellow urine
→ thirst
→ headache

When dehydration is more severe:
→ reduced concentration
→ child displays a tendency to become easily fatigued and exercise feels harder.

Children should drink 6–8 (200ml) glasses of water, or equivalent, a day under normal circumstances. After exercise they should drink until they no longer feel thirsty and then have another 200ml on top of that.

What to drink: For normal rehydration, water is fine and has the added benefit of being free from calories and artificial additives. Very sugary drinks are not generally the best way of rehydrating children (except for older children involved in prolonged intense sport).

If dehydration is severe, both fluid and body minerals (electrolytes) will have been lost and need to be replaced. An isotonic drink, which contains a higher concentration of carbohydrate (up to 8g per 100ml) as well as sodium, could be the answer.

See also: Drinks p153, Water p218.

Diabetes

Diabetes – or diabetes mellitus, to give it its full name – is a disease caused by insufficient insulin, the hormone which regulates blood glucose levels and helps the glucose to be utilized by the body. When insulin is lacking or unable to function properly, blood sugar levels rise and this can be very dangerous. Untreated diabetes can damage the organs, including the heart and kidneys.

There are two types of diabetes. Type 1 (insulin-dependent/IDDM) more commonly occurs in children and young adults, and while there is no cure, the condition is managed with regular insulin injections. Type 2 (non-insulin dependent/ NIDDM) diabetes is on the increase across the Western world. Experts believe this is because of our Western diet, increasing incidence of obesity and lack of exercise. Weight gain and lack of activity appear to produce what is known as 'insulin resistance' meaning that although the body produces insulin, it isn't sufficient – because of the amount of fatty tissue – and there is reduced sensitivity to the insulin that is produced.

Children suffering from diabetes will display some or all of the following signs:
→ Increased thirst
→ Frequent urination
→ Excessive tiredness
→ Possible blurred vision
→ Possible skin problems

Maintaining a reasonable body weight and taking regular exercise are the main ways to control or avoid NIDDM. The diet should be healthy and balanced, low in total fat and sugars. Meals should be regular and high-sugar snacks should be avoided as they tend to make the blood sugar levels fluctuate. A diet containing plenty of foods low on the Glycaemic Index can help maintain even blood sugar levels.

All children with either type of diabetes should be monitored by their doctor and given personal lifestyle and dietary advice. In Type 2 diabetes, research shows that, with careful diet and activity, insulin sensitivity can be restored to a large extent.

How to avoid type 2 diabetes? Apart from watching weight and taking enough exercise, research shows that a general healthy diet including plenty of fruit and vegetables, vitamin E and oily fish or fish oil capsules, can help to prevent insulin resistance.

See also: Obesity p189 for information on Glycaemic Index.

Dietary fibre

The more scientific name for dietary fibre is non-starch polysaccharides (NSPs). These NSPs consist of parts of the plant cell walls, such as cellulose and pectin, which are not easily absorbed within the digestive system but are nevertheless important in the diet.

NSPs are divided into insoluble fibre and soluble fibre. Insoluble fibre consists mainly of cellulose and is found in all plant matter. It adds bulk to stools, speeds the passage of food through the digestive system and is linked with prevention of bowel cancer, constipation and irritable bowel syndrome. Whole grains are a valuable source of insoluble fibre.

Soluble fibre – pectins, beta-blucans, arabinose and others – is found in highest quantities in fruits, pulses, oats, barley and rye. Soluble fibre is particularly linked with reducing LDL blood cholesterol levels and in controlling blood sugar levels. It slows the emptying of the stomach and thus can help prevent hunger and can be useful for weight control. It adds softness to the stools.

Dietary fibre and children

Very young children don't need a lot of dietary fibre as their stomachs and appetites are small and they may not take in enough calories on a high-fibre diet. But from school age onwards, a diet containing adequate fibre is important.

For children prone to overweight, fibre is especially important as high-fibre foods help a child to feel full more quickly during a meal and delay hunger returning after a meal.

Only plant foods contain fibre – meat, fish, dairy produce and eggs don't. In general, pulses, whole grains, fruit and dried fruit are the best sources of fibre. Children should get their fibre naturally from food, rather than having it added in the form of supplements or bran. Raw bran can inhibit the absorption of minerals, including calcium and iron.

It is vital to drink enough fluids with a high-fibre diet, as the fluid mixes with the fibre and waste matter to bulk out stools. Without sufficient water, fibre can't function effectively and increasing fibre in the diet without enough fluid intake can lead to constipation.

See also: Carbohydrates p144, Constipation p148.

Dried fruits

Dried fruits are a concentrated source of sugars, which is why they can be high in calories, and many are high in fibre. Although they have lost all their vitamin C in the drying process, they are an excellent source of potassium, most are a good source of iron and all contain some calcium – figs being a fairly rich source. Some dried fruits, especially figs and prunes, have a laxative effect. Prunes (dried plums) are rich in the antioxidant ferulic acid and other anti-cancer phytochemicals.

Dried fruits count towards the 'five a day' portions of fruit and vegetables although only one portion a day should count. They make a good alternative to sweets and a pleasant high-energy between-meal snack.

Many dried fruits are a good addition to rice and pasta salads, as well as coleslaw and other salads. And dried fruits can easily be reconstituted by simmering in water or juice (no added sugar needed), and then make a good addition, hot or cold, to breakfast yoghurt, or as a hot winter pudding with custard or Greek yoghurt. If you purée prunes after simmering, they can be used in cakes and bakes to add bulk and sweetness instead of some of the fat and sugar.

Many dried fruits, especially of the 'no-need-to-soak' variety, contain preservatives such as sulphur. If your child eats dried fruit, such as apricots, regularly it is probably worth buying organic, which is preservative-free – the fruit is a less appetizing colour but the taste is excellent.

Drinks

Milk is the most important drink for babies and most young children. It is rich in protein, a major source of calcium and contains valuable B vitamins. Water is the ideal drink to supplement milk in a child's diet. It is thirst quenching, helps to keep the digestive system in healthy working order, and has the advantage over most soft drinks that it is free from sugar (and acid).

Fruit juices and smoothies are beneficial for children as they are high in vitamin C and other vitamins and minerals. A child who is reluctant to eat fresh fruit may find fruit juices quite acceptable. Yoghurt drinks are another healthy option. These contain calcium and other vitamins and minerals; they may also contain probiotics.

Carbonated drinks contain carbonated water, either sugar or artificial sweeteners ('diet' versions), colourings, flavourings, preservatives and some form of acid to balance the sweetness. Most fruit squashes also contain a range of artificial additives and are high in sugar and/or artificial sweeteners. Studies indicate that a high intake of sugary drinks is a significant contributory factor towards the growing incidence of overweight and obesity in children.

There is also concern that regular use of these drinks (and fruit juice) may lead to tooth decay. Apart from the sugar, they contain acids which can spoil tooth enamel if left in contact over time – for example, if a child is allowed to sip a can or drink over a long period and this behaviour is repeated regularly.

Carbonated drinks – and squashes – are also a source of a variety of artificial additives, such as E number colourings, flavourings and preservatives, which may be a causative factor in hyperactive behaviour (or ADHD) in some children, and may be a source of food allergy.

There is no doubt that drinking water regularly is a healthier alternative for children than carbonated drinks and squashes. Good-quality drinking water should be available to all children – at home, nursery and school.

See also: ADHD p134, Behavioural Problems p139, Bone Health p141, Drinks p153, Food Additives p159, Food Allergies p162.

Dyslexia and dyspraxia

Dyslexia is a disorder in which the sufferer has specific problems in learning to read and write in relation to general ability or IQ. Problems with arithmetic and reading music are also common.

With dyspraxia, the sufferer has difficulty with physical co-ordination, including hand-eye co-ordination and tasks such as shoelace tying or getting dressed. Clumsiness is typical and there may be difficulty with organization, poor memory and temper tantrums.

Both are linked with ADHD and autism. Up to 50% of children with dyslexia or dyspraxia may also have ADHD, indeed the boundaries between these conditions are unclear.

There is some evidence to indicate that both dyslexia and dyspraxia may be improved in some children by supplementation with highly unsaturated fatty acids, particularly the fish oils DHA and EPA and possibly with GLA (evening primrose oil). Deficiencies or imbalances of these key fatty acids, which are crucial to brain development and function, may contribute to both the predisposition and the developmental expression of dyslexia and dyspraxia, as well as ADHD and autism. These fatty acids matter to everyone, but they seem particularly crucial for individuals predisposed to these kinds of specific learning difficulties.

Some typical signs of fatty acid deficiency to look out for are thirst, frequent urination, rough or dry skin (particularly on the upper arms and legs), dry hair, a tendency towards allergies, eczema and hay fever, sensitivity to light, and sleep problems.

Although the body can, in theory, manufacture the highly unsaturated fatty acids itself, lifestyle factors can inhibit this and supplements may be necessary. Diets high in saturated fats and trans fats can 'block' the conversion of certain essential fats into the longer-chain highly unsaturated fats. Zinc deficiency and caffeine can do the same. The conversion can also be hindered in people with diabetes and allergic conditions, as well as children under stress.

Eating tips for children with dyspraxia
(Dyspraxia Foundation UK)

→ Let the child sit down to eat where possible.
→ Use a damp towel under plates to stop them moving about.
→ Don't fill cups too full.
→ Provide a flexible straw with a drink to prevent spilling.

See also: ADHD p134, Autism p138, Behavioural Problems p139, Diabetes p151, Eczema p155, Essential Fatty Acids p156, Fats and Oils p157, Food Allergies p162.

E NUMBERS
see Food Additives

Eczema

Also known as atopic eczema, or dermatitis, eczema affects up to a fifth of children (often by the time they are a year old), but 60–70% are clear of the disease by the time they are 16.

Eczema is an inflammatory skin condition that causes hot, dry and itchy skin, which may break and even bleed. It is linked with asthma and other allergic conditions, and is common in children with dyslexia and related disorders. It is thought to be an allergic condition in which the immune system overreacts and produces IgG antibodies. An important factor is believed to be genetic predisposition.

Several environmental factors may trigger eczema, including house dust mites, pollen, air pollution, pets and others. Sometimes it's a symptom of food allergy – 10% of cases are thought to be caused by food allergy or intolerance, and this is more likely in babies.

Common food allergens linked to eczema are cows' milk, eggs, citrus fruits, chocolate, food colourings, peanuts and groundnut (peanut) oil. And the food eaten by a mother during pregnancy may affect the likelihood of her child developing eczema after birth.

If your child has eczema, see your doctor. If you feel that a food allergy may be triggering it, mention this to the doctor, who should arrange for your child to have tests done by a dermatologist. If this proves to be the case, it will be necessary to avoid the trigger foods.

There is evidence that supplementation with long-chain essential fatty acids can help minimize the symptoms of eczema. Omega-3s, such as those found in oily fish (DHA and EPA), and to a lesser extent the long-chain omega-3 GLA (evening primrose oil) have been shown to help a significant percentage of people in tests. These EFAs probably work because they have an anti-inflammatory effect. Supplements of 1,000mg a day of omega-3s and 300mg GLA are worth a try as they won't do any harm, but effects may not show for several weeks. In order for these fatty acids to be given a chance to work, the child's overall diet needs to be moderately low in saturated and trans fats, which will otherwise block their work. It is also worth ensuring that the child has optimum levels of vitamins A, C and E in their diet – these are all important for healthy skin and can aid healing.

If you are pregnant…

Research has suggested that much can be done while your baby is still in the womb to minimize his or her chances of getting atopic eczema and other allergies.

→ Eat foods rich in vitamin E.

→ Avoid eating those foods that most commonly produce allergic reactions in children (see left).

→ Consider taking a daily probiotic. One study showed that women given the probiotic supplement lactobacillus GG while pregnant had children who were 50% less likely to have atopic eczema at age 2.

See also: Food Allergies p162.

Eggs

Eggs are a good source of protein, vitamins B, A, D and E, and the minerals iron and zinc. To aid absorption of these valuable minerals, encourage your child to have a vitamin C-rich food or drink, such as orange juice, with an egg meal or snack. Eggs are higher in fat than you might imagine – over 50% of their total calories are in the form of fat, and over 20% of this is saturated. They are also high in cholesterol. But, if your child likes eggs, there is no reason why they shouldn't be included in the diet regularly. My advice is that you can give older children up to 6 eggs per week.

The shell colour of an egg doesn't make any difference to its nutritional value, neither does the colour of the yolk. A deep yellow yolk may be the result of the laying hen having been fed a diet that includes the food colorant canthaxanthin (E161g), high levels of which may have negative side-effects. Organic egg yolks are often quite pale.

Salmonella is still present in some eggs in the UK, so they can, potentially, be a cause of food poisoning. Always cook eggs thoroughly and avoid dirty eggs, any with cracked shells, and those that are out of their date stamp.

Use the following egg safety guidelines:
→ **Babies 6 months or under** – no egg at all.
→ **Babies 6–9 months** – can now be given hard-cooked egg yolk, but egg white and undercooked egg yolk should be avoided.
→ **Infants 9–12 months** – can be given well-cooked egg white as well as yolk now.

→ **Children under school-age** – should not be given raw or partially cooked eggs.

See also: Food Additives p159, Food Poisoning p166, Food Safety p167.

Essential fatty acids

There are two fats that are essential for the maintenance of health and development in humans that cannot be manufactured in the body, both of which are polyunsaturated fats. One is linoleic acid, which is the 'head' of the omega-6 group of fatty acids and which can be converted in the body into the omega-6s 'lower down' in the group. The other is alpha-linolenic acid, which is the 'head' of the omega-3 group of fatty acids, which can be converted in the body into the omega-3s 'lower down' in this group.

Within the omega-3 group are two special 'long-chain' fatty acids – eicosapentaenoic acid (EPA) and docosahexaenoic acid (DHA). Although, in theory, these can be made in the body from alpha-linolenic acid, it is thought that this process may be blunted by various factors, and research has shown that if EPA and DHA are eaten regularly there are significant health benefits. Adequate intake of these fatty acids is linked with improved brain power and concentration, protection against heart disease and the maintenance of a healthy blood cholesterol profile, while also helping to minimize the effects of eczema, asthma, food allergies, dyslexia and dyspraxia, autism and behavioural problems such as attention deficit hyperactivity disorder (ADHD).

It is also thought that the balance of intake of omega-6s and omega-3s is important – most children get too much omega-6s in their diets and not enough omega-3s.

The main sources of the omega-3 group (via alpha-linolenic acid) and of EPA and DHA are oily fish, such as sardines, mackerel, trout, tuna, kippers, herrings and salmon. Fresh (rather than canned) fish is the best source as most of the EPA and DHA are lost in the canning process. For vegetarians and vegans the main non-fish source of omega-3 oils is linseed (flax seed) oil, although walnuts and walnut oil also contain good amounts.

The main sources of the omega-6 group, via linoleic acid, are nuts (especially pine nuts and almonds), seeds (like sesame, pumpkin and sunflower seeds) and vegetable oils (such as sunflower, corn, sesame and walnut oils).

See also: ADHD p134, Asthma p137, Behavioural Problems p139, Brain Power p141, Dyslexia and Dyspraxia p154, Eczema p155, Fats and Oils (below), Fish p159.

FATIGUE
see Lethargy

Fats and oils

Up to the age of 5, fat should account for around 40% of calorie intake. Thereafter, there are no specific recommendations for children in the UK, but a maximum of 30–35% of calories is the general guideline.

Fat contains 9 calories per gram and, as such, is the most concentrated energy provider in the diet, since protein contains only 4 calories per gram and carbohydrate 3.75 calories per gram. Any surplus fat in the diet that isn't needed for energy is easily stored as body fat, so it is wise to limit fat intake to avoid excess weight gain.

All children need some fat in their diets, not least because it is the source of the fat-soluble vitamins A, D, E and K, and as the polyunsaturated fats group contains the essential fatty acids, which are vital for health.

Fats (or fatty acids, as they are properly known) can be divided into three main groups: saturated fats, monounsaturated fats and polyunsaturated fats.

Saturated fats: Saturated fats tend to be hard at room temperature. A high intake is linked with increased risk of heart and circulatory diseases, as saturates appear to encourage the formation of LDL cholesterol plaques in the arteries, and the consensus of opinion is that it is prudent to begin restricting the amount of these fats in the diet early in life. Saturated fats are found in greatest quantity in animal fats – e.g. fatty cuts of meat, suet, butter, lard, full-fat cheeses, cream, and products made with these.

A diet high in saturated fat can also block the work of the long-chain polyunsaturated fatty acids. Studies indicate that most children eat much more than the recommended level of saturated fat (10% of total energy intake).

Monounsaturated fats: These fats tend to be liquid at room temperature and partially solid when refrigerated. Found in highest quantities in olive oil, rapeseed and groundnut oil, avocados and nuts, they are, however, present in moderate amounts in most fat-containing foods. These fats are linked with lower incidence of heart disease.

Polyunsaturated fats: These are liquid at room temperature and when cold, and are contained in high amounts in many seed, grain and nut oils. They can be divided into two groups – the omega-6s (N6s) and omega-3s (N3s). At the head of each of these groups are the two essential fatty acids, linoleic acid (N6) and alpha-linolenic acid (N3), which everyone needs in their diets, albeit in small amounts.

Polyunsaturates tend to lower 'bad' LDL blood cholesterol levels, but they also have some negative attributes. Polyunsaturated oils easily oxidize, for example when used in cooking at high temperatures, and this produces high levels of free radicals in the body (see Antioxidants, page 135). A high intake of polyunsaturates also increases the requirement for vitamin E in the diet.

To minimize oxidization, polyunsaturated oils should always be stored in a cool, dark storecupboard, used up relatively quickly and not reused for cooking. Oils with a higher monounsaturated content are more suitable for cooking at high temperatures.

The average level of total polyunsaturates in children's diets is about right, but the bulk of the intake is in the form of omega-6s. The ratio of omega-3s (N3s) to omega-6s (N6s) should increase, and the intake of the highly unsaturated fatty acids, EPA and DHA should also increase, as these have important health benefits (see Essential Fatty Acids, page 156). A diet low in saturated fat can also help the work of the long-chain polyunsaturates.

Trans Fats: Trans, or hydrogenated, fats are polyunsaturated fats which are hardened during food processing so that they will be solid at room temperatures, for example in the production of hard margarine, biscuits and cakes. Research suggests that trans fats may even be more damaging to health than saturated fats. Children who eat a lot of processed foods are likely to be consuming a lot more trans fats than is recommended.

Manufacturers are not currently obliged to reveal the trans fat content in foods and these fats may be hidden on nutrition labels within total fats or within polyunsaturated totals. You can tell if a product contains trans fats, however, by reading the ingredients list, where they are usually termed 'hydrogenated fats'. The higher up the list this comes, the more trans fats the product contains.

See also: ADHD p134, Antioxidants p135, Asthma p137, Behavioural Problems p139, Brain Power p141, Dyslexia and Dyspraxia p154, Eczema p155, Essential fatty acids p156, Food Allergies p162, Obesity p189.

Fever

Fever in a child is a symptom of infection, and not an illness in itself. It is characterized by a high temperature and, usually, flushing. Call your doctor if your child has a high fever. A child with fever should drink plenty of fluids, preferably cool, and is unlikely to want to eat much while the fever is high.

See also: Convalescence p149, Illness, feeding during p180.

FIBRE

see Dietary Fibre

Fish

Cod and other white fish are good sources of low-fat protein, B vitamins and minerals, notably iodine, selenium and potassium.

Oily fish, such as salmon, herrings, mackerel, pilchards and– to a slightly lesser extent – fresh tuna, is much higher in fat but still low in saturated fat and high in the long-chain omega-3 (N3) oils EPA and DHA, linked with a whole range of health benefits, such as protection from heart disease, alleviation of asthma and eczema, and even improvements in children's behaviour and performance at school. Children should eat a portion of oily fish a week to get enough omega-3s in their diet, plus at least one portion of white fish.

The UK Food Standards Agency doesn't advise eating more than this as the benefits may be outweighed by consuming toxins such as mercury and other dioxins found in oily fish. Levels of these environmental pollutants have mainly fallen over the past 10 years and they vary in fish. For example, the dioxin level in trout is low, while in herring it is quite high. The advice for pregnant or breast-feeding women, or women trying to become pregnant, is that oily fish can be eaten twice a week.

Swordfish, marlin and shark have been found to contain higher levels of mercury and are not recommended for children. Smoked fish, such as kippers, may be potentially carcinogenic, so consumption of this too should be limited. There have been some recent concerns by consumer groups over levels of contaminants, antibiotic residues, and food colourings in farmed salmon.

Shellfish is low in fat and high in protein, vitamins and minerals, but prawns, in particular, are very high in sodium, and shellfish is one of the foods most likely to provoke allergic reaction in children.

When to start children on fish:

→ **Babies under 6 months** – shouldn't be given any fish.
→ **From 6–9 months** – you can offer white fish, such as coley and cod, but no oily fish.
→ **From 9–12 months** – try offering small amounts of oily fish, such as tuna.
→ **After 1 year** – a variety of fish can be offered, but children should not be fed swordfish, marlin or shark.

Use the following fish safety guidelines:

→ Make sure all fish and shellfish is very fresh and cook soon after purchase.
→ For small children, flake all fish carefully and make sure there are no bones in it.
→ If there may be bones in fish, warn older children to look out for them.
→ Go carefully when offering small children shellfish. Make sure it is well cooked, and remember that this is a common allergen.
→ Don't give children raw fish.

See also: Essential fatty acids p156, Fats and Oils p157, Food Safety p167.

Food additives

Many of the foods and drinks manufactured primarily to appeal to children contain additives, most of which add nothing to the nutritional value of the food. Indeed, there is often a long list of these additions – colorants, preservatives, flavourings, flavour enhancers and many more. Sadly, there is also a strong link between additives and food with a poor nutritional profile. Most foods containing additives are also high in the exact nutrients that many children need to eat less of – total fat, saturated fat, sugar and/or sodium (salt). The implication, according to The Food Commission, is that 'additives are being used to sell just those foods of which children should be eating less.' In theory, additives are only allowed in foods according to EU law if there is a 'technological need' for them, but one virtual loophole allows 'organoleptic qualities' to be improved. This means that the sensual quality of the food may be enhanced by their addition and this includes the colour (bright-red or orange to drinks, for example, to make the drinking experience 'more attractive' for children).

A word about flavourings...

Artificial food flavourings make up a large proportion of the additives we consume. They are controlled by different laws to other food additives and they don't have E numbers. Ingredients lists on food labels will indicate if flavourings have been used, but individual flavourings won't necessarily be named.

Why are additives used?

Additives are used to enhance flavour, colour, texture and/or appearance, to help prevent a product deteriorating, to keep consistency in manufactured foods and sometimes to help the manufacturing process.

Additives and health

There are regulations governing the use of additives and the amounts present in our foods are considered to be safe to consume by the authorities. The UK Food Standards Agency, says, for example, 'Giving an additive an E number means that it has passed safety tests and has been approved for use... EU legislation requires most additives to be labelled clearly in the list of ingredients either by name or by an E number. It is illegal in the UK to put anything into food that will injure health.' Many lovers of fresh and natural food feel that the use of additives is unnecessary.

It is true that some additives are 'normal ingredients in foods' – for example, the antioxidants used to stop fats going rancid may be vitamin C (ascorbic acid) and vitamin E (alpha-tocopherol) – on the other hand, they may be BHA, BHT, or one or more of several other non-natural additives. Other 'additives' include salt, sugar and its many variants, such as glucose and corn syrup.

However, a high percentage of additives are not normally found in food, nor are they natural. And one of the main problems is that – with the increasing reliance on highly processed, fast foods, ready foods and convenience meals for our children – the long-term cumulative effect of these high intakes of additives is still unknown. 'Safe levels' of additives are worked out scientifically, based on the assumption that an adult or child averages a certain amount of that particular type of drink or food in a day. They do not take into account the possible consumption of other processed items containing the same additive.

There is plenty of research to show that additives may, indeed, be linked with health problems in our children. Elsewhere in this section, you will find that additives may cause or exacerbate ADHD, behavioural problems, allergies and asthma. Sometimes additives thought to be safe are later found not to be – for example, in 2003 the EU curtailed the use of the colorant canthaxanthin (E161g), widely used in farmed salmon and egg production, because a high intake of this compound is linked with eyesight problems.

The following is a list of additives that have caused the most reported problems in children and therefore seem most likely to provoke a reaction. All of these are legal and declared safe!

Additives most likely to cause a problem:
Colours:
→ Tartrazine (E102)
→ Sunset yellow (E110)
→ Carmoisine (E122)
→ Ponceau 4R (E124)
Preservatives:
→ Sodium benzoate (E211)
→ Other benzoates (E210–219)
→ Sulphides (E220–228)
→ Nitrates and nitrites (E249–E252)
Flavour enhancers:
→ Monosodium glutamate and other glutamates (E621–623)
Antioxidants:
→ E310–312, E320, E321

Helping your children to avoid additives
While many children consume additives without any noticeable side-effects, the long-term cumulative effect is unknown, and most food additives add nothing of benefit to our children's diets. Here are some simple strategies to cut back on your children's intake of additives:
→ Go for natural unprocessed foods as much as possible. These will have a shorter shelf-life, so make sure they are fresh, store them in optimal conditions and always use by the 'best before' date.
→ Try to do more home cooking – additives are rarely needed in home-cooked food.
→ When buying convenience foods, go for quality and choose frozen or canned foods to cut down on preservative content.
→ Avoid foods known often to contain high levels of additives, particularly colourings, which seem to be more likely to affect children – brightly coloured soft drinks, sweets, packet desserts, processed cakes and biscuits, for example.
→ If a food or drink looks too vividly coloured to be true, it probably is. Even meat may be colour-enhanced to make it look more attractive. Nitrites are present in many preserved meats, such as bacon. These not only help to prevent bacteria but can also make the meat appear more red.
→ Read the labels – the longer the list of E numbers or chemical-sounding ingredients, the more additives that product contains.

See also: ADHD p134, Asthma p137, Behavioural Problems p139, Food Allergies p162, Food Labelling p164, Processed Foods p199, Ready Meals p202.

Food allergies

Food allergies and food intolerance seem to be on the increase and children are at a much higher risk of having or developing an allergy or intolerance than adults. About 5% of children under the age of 4 have a food allergy, as opposed to only 1-2% of adults.

Food allergy

True food allergy is an adverse – and often immediate – reaction to a food or drink, caused by an overreaction by the body's immune system to something in that food or drink. A true allergy can be confirmed by testing. Typical reactions are: swollen lips, itchy mouth, hives, vomiting, diarrhoea, stomach ache, itchy rash (eczema), coughing or wheezing, runny nose, headache.

The most common foods which produce an allergic reaction in children are: cows' milk, peanuts (groundnuts), other nuts, eggs, soya milk and soya products, wheat, sesame seeds, fish and shellfish. However, many other foods may cause allergy. There is some evidence that some food additives can also cause allergic reactions.

Peanut allergy or other nut allergy is one of the most common – and fastest-growing – allergies in children and it is one of the few that is usually life-long. Research suggests that peanut allergy can be caused by the use of baby and child skin creams containing peanut oil, and there is even some evidence that peanut allergy may be caused by consuming soya milk or formula (both soya and peanuts are members of the legume family). Once a nut allergy is diagnosed, the only 'cure' is to avoid nuts and nut traces throughout life. Many food allergies are, however, outgrown by the time a child is of school age, or if not, by their teens, although some allergies are never outgrown. Coeliac disease is an allergy to gluten in grains and this has its own A-Z entry.

Food intolerance

Food intolerance is perhaps less serious, and less easy to diagnose. It is a non-allergic reaction to food, not involving the immune system, with less predictable outcomes and the symptoms may be milder. It may be caused by a defect in how the body processes food, but there are other possible explanations.

One well-known form of food intolerance is lactose intolerance. Sufferers lack a special enzyme (lactase) in the body, which breaks down the sugars (lactose) in milk and dairy products, causing bloating, discomfort and diarrhoea, and, possibly, failure to thrive or grow properly. Some children who are lactose intolerant may be able to take goats' milk and possibly hard cheeses; others can take skimmed but not whole milk, while others use soya products instead. Lactose intolerance varies in the strength of its symptoms and may go undiagnosed. It is often outgrown.

If you think your child might have a food allergy or intolerance: The only course of action is to take him or her to your doctor and get the right tests done, and then to see the dietitian for professional advice. Some nutritionists recommend exclusion diets to try to pinpoint allergies or intolerance but these are not easy to carry out and the results may be confusing. Childhood allergies can be hard to diagnose and cope with – get professional help!

If you know your child has a food allergy: A child who has already had an immediate reaction to a particular food should not eat that food again or even, in some cases, come into contact with that food. A subsequent reaction could be more serious than the first one (see Anaphylactic Shock below). You need be given antidote medication – antihistamine and adrenaline – which should be with the child at all times in case of emergency.

Anaphylactic shock

A severe and life-threatening allergic reaction to a food (or a sting or drug) which can occur after ingesting or even touching that food. Histamine and other chemicals are produced immediately in the body, the blood vessels widen and the blood pressure drops. Symptoms include red weals, rash or hives, wheezing and shortness of breath due to the airways being constricted, and swelling of the tongue and/or throat. This is a medical emergency and the antidote medication should be given immediately and a doctor or ambulance summoned. For further information contact the Anaphylaxis Campaign (see Contacts, page 219).

MMR and eggs

The MMR (combined measles, mumps and rubella) vaccine is egg-based and if a child has a known allergy to eggs the vaccine should be given in a hospital setting. It is best to discuss the issue with your doctor.

Preventing and coping with food allergy and intolerance

Children who have one or more parents with food allergies, asthma or eczema, are more at risk, as there is a genetic influence. Breast-feeding may offer protection against allergy, but for 'atopic' women, who themselves have an allergy, asthma or eczema, it is advisable during pregnancy to avoid eating the foods most likely to cause allergy, such as peanuts, as this can sensitize the baby in the womb. They should also avoid these foods while breast-feeding.

Babies and small children from atopic families should also not be given the known allergenic foods when they are small. Indeed, certain foods should be avoided by all infants. For more information, see Allergies and Infants (page 22).

At present, there is no cure for allergies and intolerance except to avoid the offending food(s). It is therefore important to read food labels carefully and to get advice on feeding your child a proper balanced diet while excluding the problem food(s).

For many allergic children, a balanced diet isn't a problem, as the allergen food may be something that isn't commonly eaten (e.g. shellfish or sesame seeds). But, excluding such foods as wheat, milk and milk products, soya and nuts from a diet can be difficult as these are either staple foods, or present in many manufactured foods under various guises. Nut and soya allergy sufferers probably have the hardest time, as nut traces may be present in many foods and soya is a 'hidden ingredient' of many processed foods. See list of foods that may contain nuts (page 189).

The EU and the UK Food Standards Agency are currently strengthening the food labelling rules to help sufferers recognize foods they should avoid. Eating out and takeaways can be a problem and the FSA is continuing to raise awareness of the problem amongst caterers. Food manufacturers and supermarkets will normally provide lists of foods containing particular ingredients so that these can be avoided, while further help can be obtained from the British Allergy Foundation.

See also: Allergies and Infants p22, Peanuts and Food Allergies p56, Asthma p137, Coeliac Disease p147, Eczema p155, Food Additives p159, Food Labelling (below), Milk p184, Nuts p188, Contacts p219.

Food labelling

Reading food labels, particularly those on products aimed at children, is something of a minefield. The information you want is usually there – but it may take some interpreting.

The banner label (front of pack)

This is the manufacturer's shop window and he will do his best to sell this product to you – or your child – by how it looks and what it says. Although in the UK the Food Safety Act 1990 made it an offence to 'falsely describe a food or to mislead as to its nature, substance or quality', there is still room for manoeuvre. Here are the main things to watch out for:

Drink descriptions: Watch out for 'juice drink' (usually in small print) – a juice drink need contain only 10% real juice and will usually have a high content of sugar or sweeteners, colourings and flavourings. 'Pure fruit juices' that may be kept in the chilled counter are often made from concentrated juices with origin unspecified – not at all fresh!

Flavour descriptions: A dessert described as, for example, 'cherry-flavoured' probably contains no real cherry or cherry derivative at all. Flavours like these are nearly always artificially created. Even descriptions like 'with real cherries!' can be misleading – the 'real cherry' content may be minimal.

Hidden ingredients: There may be ingredients in a product which aren't immediately apparent from the front of the pack. For example, a chicken stock cube might actually contain beef! There are hundreds of other instances of this. Vegetarians, in particular, need to be wary of items such as gelatine in yoghurts or animal rennet in cheeses – look for products with a 'suitable for vegetarians' symbol and read the ingredients list carefully.

Meat descriptions: Manufacturers of meat products, such as sausages, burgers and pies, are now required to give information about the type of meat their products contain – for example, meat fat, skin and connective tissue are listed separately from the lean flesh meat, and the presence of mechanically recovered meat must be revealed. Cheaper products are likely to contain less 'real' meat. A lot of meat also contains a significant amount of water – pumped in to bulk up the weight. Frozen fish (such as prawns) also contains added water.

Percentage of ingredients: The pictures on food packages must not mislead, for example by showing fresh fruit on a pot of yoghurt, which derives its flavour solely from artificial flavourings. However, a chicken pie, for example, may contain less chicken than the photograph on the pack suggests. Check the ingredients list to see how far down the list the chicken actually comes (see page 166).

Health claims and inferences: Many products give the impression that they are somehow healthier than other similar products, perhaps by their name and/or the way the pack is illustrated. They might also be described as 'natural' or 'wholesome', and/or by banners saying 'reduced-fat' or 'reduced-sugar' and so on. Fat-reduced products may not be all that low in fat at all, and may also contain as many calories as their ordinary counterparts (because other ingredients, such as sugar, are increased). Reduced-sugar items may be high in artificial sweeteners.

Also watch out for claims such as 'free from artificial colourings' – a look at the ingredients list may well reveal that the product is NOT free from artificial preservatives, flavourings, and so on!

To claim that a product is high in, or a rich source of, certain vitamins or minerals, it must provide at least 50% of a day's recommended intake of that vitamin or mineral in a single serving.

The 'low in fat' scam: One often-used ploy to make a product appear very low in fat when really it isn't, is to use the 'xx% fat' claim. Let's say a chipped potato product is bannered as containing 'only 5% fat'. This means that 5% of the weight of the chips – i.e., 5g per 100g of chips – is fat. This doesn't mean that only 5% of the total calories in the chips are fat calories. Why? Because chips – and all other foods – have a high water content, which is calorie-free. Thus 5%-fat chips, which are about 60% water, will, in fact, have a fat content of about 28% of total calories. Not high, but not exactly low either!

The nutrition panel

Most products now list the amount of calories, fat, sugars, fibre and sodium/salt in them, though there is only a mandatory requirement for a product to carry a nutritional panel if it makes a nutrition or health claim on its pack. If there is a claim for either calorie content or amount of protein or carbohydrate or fat, it must have a Nutrition Panel listing the amount of each of these nutrients per 100g or product. If other claims are made (e.g., 'high in fibre' or 'low in saturated fat') then a more detailed Nutrition Panel is required.

When reading a nutrition panel, watch out for:

→ The 100g problem – although some packs list nutrients per serving, many others don't and you then have to look at the total weight of the product, perhaps find a 'number of servings' recommendation on the pack, and work out what the actual nutrient content for a portion may be.

→ Sodium – if a pack lists the sodium content of a food, remember that this isn't the same as salt. You need to multiply sodium content by 2.5 to get the salt content (see page 204).

→ Dry weights and reconstituted weights – if buying, say, a pack of dry instant dessert mix, the nutrients listed may be for the dry weight – not for the reconstituted weight.

The ingredients list

Ingredients are listed in descending order of weight (percentage of content), so the first one listed will be that with the highest content, the last ingredient will be the smallest.

→ E numbers should be included in this list but are allowed to be listed by their actual names (e.g. tartrazine rather than E102). Ingredients of flavourings don't have to be listed individually.

→ Additives used in an ingredient forming a small part of the recipe (e.g. the sulphur dioxide used to preserve dried fruits in a currant cake) needn't be listed.

→ Sugars come in several different forms, look out for: sucrose (proper name for sugar), glucose, glucose syrup, maltose, lactose, dextrose, hydrolized starch, honey, treacle, syrup and concentrated fruit juices.

→ Trans fats are usually listed as hydrogenated fats or hardened fats.

See also: Food Poisoning (below) and Food Safety p167 for information on use-by dates, Nuts p188 for information on the labelling of products which may contain nuts or nut traces.

Food poisoning

This is more dangerous in children, as well as the elderly and the sick, whose immune systems may be weaker than the typical adult.

The main causes of food poisoning are five different types of bacteria: campylobacter, salmonella, E coli, clostridium perfringens and listeria, although fungi and viruses may also occasionally be to blame. Even small amounts of bacteria present in food can grow to harmful levels in the right environment –

warm, moist conditions. Poor food hygiene and management can also help spread the harmful bugs.

Bacteria linked to food poisoning

→ **Campylobacter** – responsible for about half of all UK cases of food poisoning, this is most likely to occur in poultry, red meat, untreated water and unpasteurized milk.

→ **Salmonella** – the second largest cause of food poisoning in the UK, this is most often caused be raw or undercooked meat, poultry or eggs, or unpasteurized milk.

→ **E coli** – responsible for an increasing number of food poisoning cases, which can be dangerous. Undercooked minced beef and unpasteurized milk are likely sources.

→ **Clostridium perfringens** is implicated in a small number of cases. Meat, poultry and many other foods may be responsible, notably those kept warm and insufficiently reheated.

→ **Listeria** cases of food poisoning are particularly dangerous for pregnant women and small children, but they are uncommon. Soft mould-ripened cheeses, pâtés and pre-packed hams are potential sources.

All the tips described in the following entry on Food Safety can greatly reduce the chances of anyone in your family getting food poisoning.

Detecting food poisoning in children: Since the bacteria that cause most food poisoning enter the body via the digestive system, most of the symptoms will be centred on this area. After a contaminated food has been eaten, symptoms may take hours – or even days – to appear, though a few hours is probably most usual.

First symptoms are often feelings of nausea followed by vomiting and generally feeling unwell. This is often followed by abdominal cramps and diarrhoea, and possibly a fever.

What to do: Many types of food poisoning bug are resistant to antibiotics and most cases clear up by themselves. However, if you are worried about your child, the symptoms last longer than a couple of days, or there is blood in the stools, take him or her to the doctor.

There is little point trying to feed the child while they are feeling, or being, sick but it is important to rehydrate them. You can buy oral rehydration solution from the chemist, or make your own by adding a pinch (1/3 tsp) salt and l tsp of sugar to 250ml water. As the child recovers, gradually start offering easily digested, plain foods, like mashed banana or mashed potato or whatever the child asks for – they usually know what they'll be able to eat.

If you think the food poisoning was caused by food eaten outside the home, you should report the incident to your local environmental health service (details can be obtained from the UK Food Standards Agency).

See also: Convalescence p149, Food Safety (below), Illness, feeding during p180, Contacts p219 for Food Standards Agency.

Food safety

To minimize the risk of food poisoning in your family, sensible food management, kitchen practice and good hygiene are all important.

Buying and storing food

Food safety begins with buying food that is as fresh as possible, and of good quality. When shopping, check 'sell by'/'use by' dates and buy those that are as far ahead of these dates as possible.

→ Check and make sure eggs aren't cracked.

→ In shops where meat and fish is sold unpacked, avoid any with a noticeable odour. Avoid minced meat which doesn't look red.

→ If doing a big shop, try to buy meat, fish and frozen foods last, so that they remain cool, pack them in cool-bags (vital in hot weather) and get them home quickly.

→ Unpack food as soon as you get home and put it away, starting with any frozen foods. Then put away all fresh meat, fish, fruit and vegetables (with the exception of potatoes) in the fridge (or freeze them, carefully wrapped and labelled, if appropriate). To avoid cross-contamination, don't store raw meats above cooked meats, and always store raw meat in a sealable container. Keep raw foods away from cooked foods. Make sure everything is well wrapped, bagged or sealed in a container. Always wash hands after handling raw foods.

→ Store eggs in the fridge – they only need an hour or two out of the fridge for recipes that require them at room temperature.

→ When freezing, keep like foods together. Vegetables are best blanched before freezing.

→ Make sure your fridge and freezer are at the correct temperature.

→ Keep dry goods like flour, grains, pasta and rice, in lidded containers in a cool dry place.

→ Use up food in date order.

→ Discard any badly dented cans or tins.

→ Clean the fridge and all food storage cupboards regularly.

Food preparation and equipment

→ Check the 'use by' date on food and discard if out of date, even by just one day.

→ Wash your hands thoroughly before starting to prepare food and after every visit to the toilet or after tasks such as emptying the bin or changing a baby's nappy.

→ Wash salads and fruit to be eaten raw.

→ Defrost all food thoroughly before cooking, unless the label says otherwise. It is essential to defrost chicken and minced meat properly.

→ Use a separate chopping board for preparing raw meat and another for other raw foods. Use a different board for preparing food that will be eaten without any further cooking.

→ After preparing raw foods, clean knives or other utensils, wash the chopping board and work surface thoroughly and always wash your hands. Wash the taps, which you will probably have touched. Use very hot water and detergent to clean everything. Dry your hands on clean kitchen paper before continuing to prepare other food. Don't dry your hands on your apron or tea towel.

→ Once raw food is prepared, don't leave it hanging around in the kitchen for long before cooking it. If cooking is to be delayed, put it in a container, cover and place in the fridge.

Cooking

→ Cook all meat thoroughly for children – especially make sure that chicken is cooked right through, with no pink juice or flesh, and make sure that burgers, sausages and other minced meat products are cooked all the way through. Proper cooking kills many bugs including salmonella and campylobacter.

→ To test that meat is cooked through, insert a clean skewer through the thickest part to check the juices run clear.

→ Cook fish and shellfish properly.

→ Make sure that eggs are well cooked for all young children and sick children.

→ Before serving any dish, check it is cooked right through to the middle and is piping hot.

→ When heating up (or cooking) a ready-made dish, follow the pack instructions, and make sure that it is fully heated or cooked through.

Storing and reheating cooked food

→ Once food is cooked, if it isn't to be eaten at once, cool it as quickly as possible and place in a sealed container in the fridge within 2 hours.

→ Don't keep cooked foods in the fridge for more than a day – either use or discard them. Pasta, rice, fish and shellfish dishes are best discarded if not eaten straight away.

→ Refrigerate leftovers immediately after the meal is finished, but not from people's plates.

→ Reheat cooked food thoroughly until it is piping hot. If microwaving food to reheat, make sure it is hot all the way through.

→ If any food doesn't smell or look right, discard it rather than take a risk.

Eating out

Over 70% of people who get food poisoning believe that it was caused by a food eaten outside the home. Indeed, the increase in fast food, café and takeaway eating is often cited as a cause of the rise in food poisoning cases. When eating out with the family, make sure the place and staff look clean and tidy, and that utensils and crockery are properly clean.

Make sure that ready-to-eat salads, cooked meats and sandwiches, and all other ready-to-eat food is well covered to avoid insects, and is kept in a chilled environment. Check that raw foods aren't displayed anywhere near cooked foods. If food is not properly cooked or if it is supposed to be served hot and isn't, don't eat it. And do check that your children's food is properly cooked – don't rely on them to tell you.

Barbecues

All children love a barbecue, but you need to take some safety precautions in order to keep the food safe. The biggest risk to children's health is from undercooked meat and from cross-contamination – allowing raw meats or utensils, or hands that have touched raw meats, to come into contact with food that is to be eaten without cooking, or that is already cooked). Food left hanging around outdoors in heat is another danger.

Avoiding undercooked meat:
→ Make sure the barbecue is properly hot before starting to cook – the coals should be glowing with a powdery grey surface.
→ Make sure all frozen food is thoroughly defrosted before barbecuing.
→ To ensure thorough cooking, pre-cook chicken portions (in an oven preheated to 180°C/gas 4 for 25 minutes) before putting them on the barbecue. You could also use this method for large sausages and any pork meat.
→ Turn food regularly and move it around to make sure that everything gets cooked evenly.
→ Before serving, check that meat is piping hot in the middle and cooked through.

→ Discard all barbecued leftovers unless they have been taken into the house, cooled and refrigerated immediately after cooking.
Avoiding cross-contamination:
→ Always keep raw and cooked meat on separate plates and never put cooked meat on a plate that has been used for raw meat.
→ Don't let raw meat come into contact with food that isn't to be cooked – e.g. burger buns.
→ Don't let raw meat come into contact with cooked or partly cooked meat on the barbecue.
→ Keep separate utensils for raw and cooked foods.
→ Wash hands between handling raw meat and serving non-cook foods.
Other tips:
→ Keep prepared salads and sauces covered in a cool place in the house until just before you serve them, to avoid bacteria build-up and contamination by insects or pets.
→ Try to have a table set aside outdoors in the shade for salads, breads, drinks, etc.
→ Don't bring out desserts until after the main barbecue has been eaten, especially ones that contain cream.

Picnics

→ Unless the picnic is to be eaten fairly soon after it has been prepared, avoid salads and sandwiches containing meat, fish or pâtés; avoid meat pasties.
→ Take food in cool-boxes or bags and don't unpack it until just before it is time to eat.
→ Take antiseptic hand wipes to use before eating. Children playing in fields and parks can easily pick up bugs and such, that may contaminate the food that they handle.

Food standards

The long-term implications of food standards issues, such as pesticide residues and genetically modified foods in our children's diets are considered here.

Residues in food

The type of intensive or factory farming that has been carried out across the Western world for many years now has brought up some pertinent safety considerations, not least of which are worries about the contamination of our food with pesticides or herbicides in plants and growth hormones and antibiotics in animals.

Of course, there are strict regulations governing the use of these chemicals, and there is regular testing to ensure that these are being obeyed. Unfortunately, samples are sometimes found to contain more than the permitted levels. For example, in the UK, pesticide levels are regularly tested in a range of vegetables, and a small percentage of items, such as lettuce and carrots, are often found to contain levels over the legal limit.

Safe plant foods: As we are being urged to eat more fruits and vegetables – most of which have been grown with the help of pesticides, herbicides and a variety of chemical fertilisers and may then have been treated with other chemicals to prolong 'freshness' or storage time – there is cause for concern. Even if residue levels are acceptable in individual items, the cumulative effect, if our children eat a lot of fruit and veg, may be more of a problem. The exception is if proper organic farming methods have been used (see Organic Foods, page 193.)

The truth is that nobody really knows the long-term effects of eating a diet containing these residues. Until we do know, it may be prudent to choose to grow or buy organic produce, or, at least, the organic versions of the more vulnerable plant foods.

Particularly vulnerable plant foods:

→ Those imported from countries outside the EU, whose growing methods are harder to trace and laws may be less strict than ours.

→ Leafy vegetables – e.g. cabbage and lettuce. Vegetables with a lot of surface area are likely to contain higher overall residue levels.

→ Carrots – residue levels in carrots tend to be higher than in many other vegetables.

→ Produce made from grains such as wheat. Grains, being small, like lettuce will tend to absorb higher levels of residue. They are also a food staple, so our children's intake is normally high.

→ Fruits and vegetables that aren't peeled. Peeling can remove a percentage of the residues – but for health reasons many parents encourage their children to eat peel, skins, and so on. Washing can also help to remove a small amount of residue.

Safe animal and dairy foods: Factory or intensive farming of our beef, pigs, poultry, eggs and dairy herds – and even of our fish – means that much of the animal produce on sale in our supermarkets contains traces of residues in their feeds. There may also be traces of growth hormones used to promote faster or larger growth, and perhaps traces of antibiotics used to contain disease and also to improve growth rates. What animals eat will also show up in their milk, flesh and organs. Again, there is little research showing the long-term effect of regularly eating these foods on our children's health, but you may prefer to minimize his or her intake.

Tips to minimize children's intake of residues:

→ Buy organic meat, eggs and dairy produce – and/or from a local source.

→ Avoid imported produce – standards of production overseas are sometimes less stringent than our own.

→ Buy lean meat and cut fat off meat when you see it – toxins tend to accumulate in fat, not lean, flesh.

→ Lamb is generally reared in a more natural way than any other of our meats.

→ Avoid factory-farmed fish, such as salmon or trout, as these may contain antibiotic residues and possibly be artificially colour-enhanced. If possible, buy fish caught by traditional methods in deep waters.

Heavy metals and industrial waste: Nutritionally, fish is good for our children and we are urged to get them to eat a portion of oily fish and at least one portion of white fish every week. The advice to eat plenty of oily fish, in particular, is tempered because it is liable to be contaminated with mercury, dioxins or PCBs, by-products of industry which have been dumped at sea or arrive there via our rivers. Dioxin levels have gradually declined in the past 10 years and overall fish is considered safe to eat, but it makes sense to exercise some caution.

White fish, which has a very low fat content, contains much lower levels of dioxins and PCBs than oily fish, as these toxins are stored in the liver and fatty tissue rather than in lean flesh. In theory, a very high consumption of oily fish by children could lead to dioxin intake beyond safe levels.

Several large non-oily fish have been found to have high levels of mercury contamination and the UK Food Standards Agency advises that children should avoid eating shark, marlin and swordfish.

Genetically modified foods

As yet, no one really knows what the long-term effects of consuming genetically altered foods or ingredients might be, but many people prefer to buy food that they know to be GM-free. It isn't feasible to eliminate GM foods entirely because the EU has set a legal 'tolerance level' enabling food that contains less than 1% GM ingredients to be declared 'GM-free'. Consequently these foods need not be labelled as containing genetically modified ingredients. Also, some products are given exempt status even if the GM ingredient is present in amounts larger than 1%. These include animal feed, oils from GM crops, lecithin and modified starches (the last two being ingredients typically added in many manufactured food processes).

Avoiding GM foods:

→ Avoid foods that have soya as an ingredient. Avoiding processed foods is the only practical way to do this, as about 70% of all processed foods contain soya in some form. About half of the world's soya crop is now genetically modified beans, which tend to be mixed with non-GM beans before distribution.

→ Avoid foods containing maize (corn) – much of the world's maize crop is now also GM.

→ Read labels carefully. When a GM content meets the legal requirements explained above, it will have to say so on the label. Much tomato purée contains modified tomatoes.

→ Buy organic – genetic modification is not allowed in foods produced to the UK Soil Association organic standard.

See also: Organic Food p193.

Fried food

Fried food has a poor profile. Oven chips, and other baked goods that taste like fried, have made the deep-fat fryer obsolete in many kitchens. If you choose to deep-fry, however, it is important to do so at the correct, constant temperature and never to overfill the pan with food as the oil temperature then drops too far and the food absorbs oil.

If using a deep-fat fryer, the oil will be prone to oxidation, which can be dangerous to health and possibly carcinogenic. To avoid oxidation, use an oil with a medium polyunsaturated fat content, such as groundnut or rapeseed oil, not an oil with a very high polyunsaturated content, such as safflower or corn oil, or blended vegetable oils. Change the oil in the pan very regularly and store it in the fridge, which also helps prevent oxidation.

For parents watching their children's fat and calorie intake, there are good alternatives to

deep-frying that are just as appealing to children's taste buds, if not more so.

Stir-frying: An ideal method for cooking a variety of vegetables – not only do children often prefer the taste, but the oil helps many of the vital phytochemicals to be more readily absorbed in the body, and also helps to retain the water-soluble vitamin C and B group. With a good-quality pan, only a small amount of oil needs to be used. For vegetables that absorb a lot of fat (e.g. aubergines), add a little stock or water rather than more fat, or turn the heat down, cover with a lid and the moisture in the vegetables will do the job itself.

Dry-frying and griddling: Many foods, including bacon, sausages and burgers, can be dry-fried or griddled with virtually no extra fat. Lightly brush the griddle or a non-stick frying pan with oil, then add the food and cook over a medium heat until the food's own fat begins to melt and run out. You can then turn the heat up higher to cook the food thoroughly.

Pan-frying: Most children enjoy a 'real' fried egg with some oven chips, and very little oil is needed. An average fried egg has an extra 3–4g fat – worth an additional 30 calories.

Shallow-frying: Food still absorbs a significant amount of fat when it is cooked in a thin layer of oil, so use this method only occasionally. Use good-quality groundnut or rapeseed oil.

Grilling: This is a healthier option to frying. Fish fingers and sausages can be grilled rather than fried and children often prefer grilled bacon. Grilled potato wedges brushed with a little olive oil make a tasty option to chips.

See also: Fats and Oils p157, Phytochemicals p195, Vegetables p212, Potato Wedges p81.

Frozen food

Food that is frozen correctly should be as nutritious as fresh food. To ensure that you make the most of frozen foods and don't compromise on food safety, there are a few guidelines you should follow:

→ Don't freeze any food that is past its sell-by date or stale. Frozen foods should be eaten within weeks (baked goods, fish, shellfish) or months (vegetables, meat) and discarded if they look dry or discoloured when you take them out of the freezer.

→ Defrost foods thoroughly before cooking, unless the label says you can cook from frozen, and cook them well.

→ Don't refreeze frozen food that has thawed, although you can refreeze frozen food which you have cooked (e.g., if you use defrosted mince to make a lasagne, you can freeze the cooked lasagne).

→ When buying frozen food, make sure that it is well frozen – avoid packs of vegetables (e.g. peas) in large lumps as this means they may have thawed and refrozen. When buying frozen foods from a shop, always use a cool-box to take them home.

Good-quality vegetables, which have been frozen within hours of picking and then properly stored, may contain more vitamin C than 'fresh' vegetables bought from a shop where they have been stored for several days (or even longer) and then kept in sunlight – both warmth and light deplete the vitamin C content of foods.

See also: Food Poisoning p166, Food Safety p167.

Fruit

All children would benefit from eating 2 or 3 portions of fruit a day, according to several reports into diet and health. One large UK study of adults who ate fruit regularly as children showed that they had less incidence of cancer in adulthood, and the World Health Organization report that around 10% of cancers in the developed world could be the result of people not eating enough fruit and vegetables. Fruit intake is also linked with less risk of other diseases. Yet, according to a UK survey of schoolchildren's diets, only 39% regularly eat fruit, and 1 in 5 have no fruit at all.

Nutrients in fruit: Most fruits are very low in fat, low in protein, low in calories and low in starch – the exception being bananas, which have a significant starch content. Most fruits are quite high in fibre and many are high in soluble fibre. Fruits are also a major source of phytochemicals – the special plant chemicals that experts believe have very important health benefits. Also, many fruits are rich in the antioxidant vitamin C and potassium.

The calorie content of fruit comes mostly from fruit sugars (called fructose). The sugar found in fruit is described as intrinsic sugar, which means that it is a natural part of the plant structure. This type of sugar, like other sugars, is associated with risk of tooth decay – but it is fruit juice that seems to pose more of a problem to teeth than whole fruits, as juice tends to be in contact with teeth and gums for longer periods than when a child is eating a portion of fruit.

Tips on serving children fruit

→ Children should have 5 portions of fruit and vegetables a day. A breakdown of 2 fruit and 3 vegetables is about right, but there is no need to stick to this to the letter.

→ To benefit from maximum vitamin C, eat fruit really fresh and always store it in the fridge. When cut, fruit immediately starts to lose its vitamin C, so only cut fruit for children immediately before they are going to eat it.

→ Offer a wide variety of different fruits to your child for maximum nutritional benefit.

→ When making fruit salad, put slices of apple and pear into the serving bowl one-quarter filled with an acidic juice (e.g. orange) to stop the fruits from going brown (oxidizing). Top up with water to serve.

→ Children who don't like chewing big lumps of fruit almost always enjoy fruit smoothies to drink, and fruit purées or coulis poured over ice cream, yoghurt, custard and so on.

→ Use fresh fruit as part of a salad platter for lunch – slices of apple go very well with cheese or ham, while oranges, mango or satsumas go well with cooked chicken.

→ Cooked fruit is often popular and although it loses some vitamin C, the other nutrients are retained. Fill cored cooking apples with a mixture of dried fruit and brown sugar, score around the circumference and bake in an ovenproof dish containing a little water at 180°C/gas 4 for 40 minutes, or until tender. Or peel, cut and cook in 1 or 2 tbsp water with a little brown sugar in a saucepan until pulpy. Slice and poach pears in fruit juice, or bake bananas in their skins to serve with yoghurt.

→ Some children are allergic to certain fruits – strawberries are a culprit and can produce symptoms such as a rash. Citrus fruits may also cause a problem. However, children often grow out of fruit allergies as they get older.

See also: The Food Pyramid p52, Berry Fruits p140, Citrus Fruits p147, Food Allergies p162, Phytochemicals p195, Teeth and Gums p209, Vegetables p212.

Fussy eating and food refusal

Fussy eating is common in pre-school children and the Royal College of Physicians (RCP) describes it as, for many, a stage of normal development. It takes several forms:

Selective eating: When a child will eat only certain foods – often quite a small range – this is termed selective eating, or extreme food faddiness. There is no particular pattern to the types of food that a child will eat – it could be only bread, jam and ice cream, or only chips, crisps and tomato ketchup – and there is a great unwillingness to try new foods.

Other children will eat only 'baby foods' with a very soft or sloppy texture (this is called 'inappropriate texture of food for age'). The child eats the foods he or she has selected happily and there are no emotional problems.

In the short term this may not be a huge health concern but, if it goes on for a long time, it may be. A very narrow range of foods can cause nutritional problems and if the foods selected are high in sugar, that may cause problems with teeth and gums. Underweight, surprisingly, is not necessarily a problem.

If you are worried, or the problem seems to have gone on for a long time, or the child seems to have restricted growth, it is wise to see your doctor, who can examine your child for health problems and may refer you to a specialist in eating problems. However, the peak age for selective eating is in the primary school years, and many children do gradually accept a wider range of foods and, eventually, eat a normal range. Experts say that trying to force the child to eat new foods, or showing extreme concern or negative emotions just makes matters worse.

Food refusal: According to the RCP, this differs from selective eating in that it is often linked with emotional problems such as worry or unhappiness, and/or food is only refused when in certain situations (e.g. at school). Once the child's worries have been identified and dealt with, the food refusal tends to go away, but you should see your doctor as professional help may be needed to help the child with his or her problems.

The RCP defines another category similar to food refusal – food avoidance emotional disorder. This seems to occur when there is chronic or acute distress in the child's life – the child may be depressed, sad, withdrawn and disinterested in food, and their refusal to eat may result in weight loss. Professional help should be sought for this problem.

Food phobia: This may occur when a child has had a particularly bad experience of eating a food. For example, he or she may have eaten something that caused choking or induced sickness. He or she may have fears about the texture or taste or odour of food, or difficulty in swallowing. The phobia results in the child refusing food, or certain foods, or certain textures. True food phobia needs treatment (cognitive therapy is often used). A visit to the doctor is a starting point. Most cases of fussy eating and food refusal do get sorted out in time, with professional help as necessary.

See also: Feeding Problems p55, Appetite Loss p136, Teeth and Gums p209, Underweight p210.

GLUTEN
see Coeliac Disease

Grains

Grains in their natural state are a good source of starchy 'complex' carbohydrate and fibre, most supply a range of minerals and some are a good source of B vitamins. They also mostly contain reasonable amounts of protein. Cereals are linked with protection from bowel and other cancers and from diverticulitis, and can also help to prevent constipation. Barley, rye and oats are a good source of soluble fibre, which helps to prevent heart disease, and they also contain phytochemicals, which have anti-cancer effects.

Refined grains – such as pearl barley and white rice – contain much less fibre, vitamins and minerals than whole grains. Wheat (and couscous, which is made from wheat), bulghar wheat, rye, barley and oats are not suitable for children with a gluten intolerance, but corn and rice are – another substitute for flours containing gluten is soya flour.

See also: Bread p142, Carbohydrates p144, Coeliac Disease p147, Dietary Fibre p152, Food Allergies p162, Phytochemicals p195.

Grapes

Grapes are higher in sugars – and, therefore, calories – than many fruits and contain less vitamin C and fibre than others. However, red grapes are rich in phytochemicals from the polyphenol group called resveratrol, which seems to be linked to protection against heart disease. Seedless grapes make a useful snack or lunch-box addition for children.

Greens, leafy

Leafy vegetables – the cabbage or cruciferous family, as well as broccoli and cauliflower, which are flower heads – are a very important group of foods with several health benefits. They are full of extraordinary plant compounds (phytochemicals) and are a particularly rich source of several minerals. They also contain good-to-excellent amounts of vitamin C, folate, carotenes and fibre.

In addition to the above nutrients, leafy greens are also a reasonably good source of iron, and its absorption is helped by the vitamin C. Spinach is rich in calcium and is also high in iron, but because of its oxalic acid content, these minerals aren't easily absorbed. The dark outer leaves of greens contain much more carotenoids than the paler leaves and hearts. Almost all greens contain a negligible amount of fat (less than 1g per 100g) and only a trace of saturates. They are all cholesterol free. Apart from sprouts, white cabbage, broccoli and cauliflower, they also contain less than 1g protein per 100g. The carbohydrate content of greens (mainly in the form of sugars), is also very low, so these vegetables are low in calories (e.g. cabbage 4g/100g).

So, it's not surprising that we were told as kids to 'eat up your greens', and are keen to get our own children to do so. The strong flavour of some greens (e.g. spinach, spring greens and Brussels sprouts) can be offputting for young children, but most children like broccoli and cauliflower. Try to serve your children several portions of 'leafy greens' a week as part of their 'five a day'.

Good sources of micronutrients

→ **Vitamin C** – sprouts, kale, spring greens
→ **Folate** – spinach, kale, sprouts
→ **Carotenoids** – kale, Savoy cabbage, spring greens, spinach
→ **Potassium** – all leafy greens
→ **Calcium** – kale, pak choi, spring greens
→ **Magnesium** – kale, broccoli

Phytochemicals in greens

Greens contain a range of plant chemicals that can protect your children's health, including:
→ Broccoli and cauliflower contain valuable glucosinolates. Broccoli has one called sulphoraphane, which inhibits cancer cells and helps stop cancer from developing.
→ Kale, spring greens and spinach are very high in the carotenoids lutein and zeaxanthin, which help keep eyes healthy and maintain good eyesight. Kale, which also contains high levels of glucosinolates (see broccoli above), contains the highest overall levels of antioxidants of all vegetables.

→ Brussels sprouts acquire their strong taste from sinigrin, a chemical that can destroy pre-cancerous cells in the body.
→ Cabbage contains indoles, a member of the glucosinolates family, which seem to block cancer-causing agents.
→ The high levels of antioxidants in all greens may also help to protect against heart disease and several other diseases.

Getting children to eat leafy greens

→ Don't overcook them. Soggy boiled greens don't taste good or feel nice in the mouth and, what's more, they lose a lot of their vitamin and mineral content into the cooking water. Steam greens over boiling water for just a few minutes until just tender and serve at once.
→ Chop or shred greens and use them along with vegetables, meat and pulses in soups and stews.
→ Cooking with a little fat or oil helps the beneficial compounds be absorbed by the body, and children usually prefer the taste. So, stir-fry in groundnut or olive oil to serve as a side vegetable, or with meat or fish as a main meal. Baked vegetables are also popular – drizzle with a little olive oil and seasoning before baking. If you give greens as part of a meal that contains fat (e.g. with a Sunday roast) this also serves the same purpose.
→ Use greens in salads – white cabbage in a coleslaw, red cabbage in a winter salad with carrot and beansprouts; pak choi or Chinese leaves (similar nutritional profile) instead of lettuce.

See also: Antioxidants p135, Minerals p185, Phytochemicals p195, Vitamins p213.

Grilled food

Grilling is a good way to lower the fat content of a variety of meats – such as lamb or pork chops, bacon, gammon, sausages and burgers – as the fat runs away from the food and is easily discarded. When grilling or barbecuing, however, care should be taken to avoid overcooking or burning the food. When lean meat (beef, lamb, pork, chicken and even fish) is cooked at high temperatures, the proteins in the meat react to form hydrocarbons which have been linked with increased risk of certain cancers. Also, when barbecuing over coals or wood, aromatic amines in the smoke may also be cancer-causing.

To minimize the risk from grilled or barbecued foods, keep the cooking heat moderate only (don't cook over coals until they are greyish and glowing). Precook large pieces of meat and just finish off on the barbecue. Serve with plenty of salad or vegetables and follow with fruit, all of which contain antioxidants to mop up harmful chemicals that may be in the grilled food.

Take special care when grilling meat for children that it is cooked all the way through and no pink flesh remains – undercooked burgers and chicken are especially dangerous.

See also: Food Safety p167, Fried Food p172.

Hay fever

It is quite common for children to suffer from seasonal allergic rhinitis, as hay fever is properly called. This allergic reaction to airborne pollens from trees and grass, when high levels of histamine are released in the body, may start as early as March (tree pollen) and continue until mid-summer. Symptoms are sneezing, runny nose, streaming eyes and, perhaps, headache, itching and inflammation of the nasal passages.

Some trials have shown that a daily supplement of 500mg vitamin C can help to reduce the severity of hay fever by reducing the levels of histamine. There is also evidence that bioflavonoids, a group of phytochemicals found in citrus fruits, onions, apples and many fruits and vegetables, can act as natural antihistamines. So a balanced diet high in fruit and vegetables seems the best line of approach to help hay fever sufferers.

See also: Asthma p137, Food Allergies p162, Phytochemicals p195.

Health foods

The term 'health food' means different things to different people. To some, it is everything that is sold in a 'health-food shop'; to others, it means organic food; to many, it is simply fresh unrefined natural foods; to some, it refers to food supplements and herbal remedies; to others, it means food that is well-balanced nutritionally.

In fact, there is no real or legal definition of a 'health food'. There is a healthy diet, which varies somewhat from individual to individual, and there are nutrient-rich foods, which may be rich in a few, or some, or very many, of all the nutrients we need for good health or body maintenance. 'Healthy eating' is sensible eating with a wide variety of different good-quality foods. And what is good quality? Fresh food, grown in a responsible way and stored to retain maximum nutrients. If cooked or processed, add that it should be cooked and/or processed in a responsible way to retain maximum natural nutrients and minimize unnecessary artificial or other additives.

Heart health

Children as young as primary school age are beginning to show early signs of, or risk factors for, heart disease – high levels of the less desirable fats in the bloodstream, obesity, and so on. Experts believe that it is never too early to start protecting the body against cardiovascular diseases and a well-balanced diet – including plenty of fruit and vegetables, whole grains, pulses and fish, as well as nuts and seeds, and possibly other items such as olive oil and garlic – can all help in this quest. The diet should also be low in saturated fats and trans fats, low in sodium and a child should not be allowed to become obese. The diet plans and recipes in this book will help you to achieve this.

For children who have a close family member (e.g. parent and/or grandparent) with cardio-vascular problems, including high blood pressure or high cholesterol, it is particularly important to lead a lifestyle which minimizes the risks – and to get regular check-ups via your doctor.

See also: Weight Issues 118, Fats and Oils p157, Obesity p189, Contacts p219 for relevant organisations.

Honey

Honey is often promoted as a healthier sweetener than sugar. It has a similar nutritional profile to sugar and although it does contain vitamins and minerals these are present in such small amounts that their contribution to the diet is minimal. However, good-quality honey does have one special property – it is a proven antibacterial and has been shown to help heal even stubborn wounds. It may also help treat mouth ulcers if applied direct to the ulcers, and may ease a sore throat if bacteria (rather than a virus) are the cause of the problem.

However, any old pot of honey won't necessarily do the trick. Research has mostly been carried out using manuka honey, a pure honey from New Zealand and Australia, which is fairly easy to find in the shops. It is likely that other pure honeys, which haven't been through too much processing, will also have an antibacterial effect. Look for honeys made by bees who frequent single types of flower, and for pure honeycomb honey.

Honey is best not given to children under 1 as it may occasionally cause infant botulism, a form of food poisoning. However, honey is a good antiseptic and is worth including in the diet of older toddlers, especially honey of good quality.

Experts haven't pinpointed the factor that gives honey such special healing powers, but it may be an ingredient or ingredients similar to the phytochemicals found in plants.

See also: Phytochemicals p195.

Hunger

If a child complains of hunger it is usually a quite natural mechanism that ensures he or she gets something to eat. Children quickly become ravenous if they spend a lot of time playing outdoors, and can eat quite amazing amounts for their size. If your child is about average weight or underweight, gets plenty of exercise and seems permanently hungry, don't worry about responding to a huge appetite, but offer good-quality foods that will provide a more sustained blood sugar level, not sugary snacks or too many crisps (see foods with a high, medium and low Glycaemic Index, page 192). Children who take little exercise and are sedentary for much of the time, but still seem to be very hungry and tend to snack while watching TV and so on, may be eating from habit, boredom or comfort. You need to help them to change their lifestyle and then the snacking habit should become less of a problem.

If your child is overweight or obese and gets very hungry, you need to be careful not to encourage unnecessary intake of calories, particularly those in the form of sweets, sugary drinks and snacks. These foods and drinks don't satisfy hunger for long – better to give your child an apple, an oat cracker with a small piece of cheese or some other foods low on the Glycaemic Index.

Children who have been unwell and are beginning to recover often develop a short-term big appetite, which is the body's way of replenishing the body fat that may have been lost. Very occasionally, a big appetite can be a sign of disease, so if you've eliminated all the other suggestions here and can't explain your child's appetite – see your doctor, who should carry out any necessary tests.

See also: Convalescence p149, Obesity p189, Underweight p210.

HYPERACTIVITY
see ADHD

Illness, Feeding During

When children have a short-term illness, such as a cold or chesty cough, they often eat less than usual. Obviously part of the reason is that being ill makes you less inclined to feel hungry. Also, sense of smell may be affected, which affects appetite. During the inactivity of illness, less calories are burnt up in any case, so eating less is a natural follow-on.

Taking all those factors into account, the best course of action is to give the child small, fairly frequent portions of food, and, as far as is sensible, give him or her what he or she feels like eating. Plenty of easy-to-eat fruit, such as seedless grapes, banana, seedless satsumas and slices of peach or pineapple are ideal. The vitamin C and plant chemicals in these fruits may help boost the immune system and speed recovery. Ice cream, Greek yoghurt and custard are all good ways to get some calcium and calories into the diet as well as soothing a sore throat.

Don't worry too much if the only savoury food they will eat is, say, soup and sandwiches, or even just bread and butter. It is surprising how many nutrients can be crammed into a bowl of homemade soup. You can also grate a little cheese on top to add more protein.

Don't be too ready to offer bland flavours – sometimes the taste buds need something a little more lively. For potent savoury flavour, try Marmite which, though too high in salt for frequent use, is a good source of B vitamins. Avoid foods very high in fat, which may cause nausea, and avoid large chunks of anything or any foods which are hard to chew or swallow.

If the appetite really has gone in the short term – don't worry. Just provide lots of fluids, such as water, diluted juices, lemon and honey in hot water, and milk, so that the child doesn't get dehydrated. For long-term illness it is best to consult a dietitian (via your doctor) for specific advice on your chid's diet.

Probiotics
If children are taking antibiotics for illness, these can destroy the good bacteria in the digestive system as well as those that are causing the symptoms. To re-colonize the gut, offer your child bio yoghurt, containing bacteria such as acidophilus and bifidus, or you can buy probiotic capsules (store them in the fridge). Research shows that probiotics can help to minimize the symptoms of both respiratory infections and diarrhoea.

See also: Convalescence p149, Honey p179.

Insomnia
Occasionally most children have a bad night's sleep and this is nothing to worry about – they tend to sleep for longer the next night. If insomnia persists for more than a couple of

nights and is bad enough to cause the child to feel overtired during the day, check that there is nothing worrying him or her – anxiety is one of the most common causes of sleeplessness for all ages, even for quite young children.

Make sure that the bed is comfortable and that the room is not too hot. Lack of exercise can cause poor sleep, so ensure that your child gets outside every day, if possible. Exercise helps relaxation and releases endorphins, which have a calming effect. A warm bath before bedtime is also a good idea.

Diet can have a considerable effect on sleep and you can help your child get a good night's sleep by giving them appropriate foods.

Food to promote a good night's sleep
→ Make sure that the child's evening meal is rich in complex carbohydrates – e.g. rice, potatoes, pasta, bread. These stimulate the production of serotonin, a chemical that has a relaxing effect on the brain. Wholegrain carbohydrates (brown basmati rice, whole-wheat pasta and wholegrain bread) keep the blood sugar levels even for longer than many highly refined carbs, as they are lower on the Glycaemic Index (see page 192). They may therefore prevent night hunger, which can keep children awake, especially those who have an early tea or supper. If supper is more than 3 hours before a child goes to bed, a bedtime snack is appropriate:
Good bedtime snacks to help sleep:
→ Digestive biscuit or oatcake with hot milk.
→ Banana sandwich on wholegrain bread.
→ Pot of whole-milk yoghurt with banana chopped in.

→ A few protein foods are rich in the amino acid tryptophan, which helps the production of serotonin. Turkey and milk both contain tryptophan and, surprisingly, bananas are another good source, although their protein content is not high.
→ Calcium is also a relaxant and a sleep-promoter, so a calcium-rich drink or snack before bedtime is a good idea. Milk is, in fact, a perfect night-time drink, as it contains carbohydrate, tryptophan and calcium, as well as B vitamins, which help tryptophan to convert to serotonin. Warm milk tends to be more soothing and comforting than cold milk, though both will do the trick.

Food to avoid to ensure a good night's sleep:
→ Anything containing the stimulant caffeine in the evening – cola drinks, chocolate, etc.
→ Hard cheese: many find that they sleep badly if they eat cheese too near to bedtime – it often seems to induce bad dreams.
→ A high-protein, low-carb evening meal, as this tends to be stimulating rather than calming.
→ A large meal just before bedtime. This can cause the digestive system to go into overdrive and disrupt sleep. A better pattern is a main meal no later than 2 hours before bed, or high tea about 3 hours before bed, followed by a small bedtime snack.

See also: Anxiety p135.

LACTOSE INTOLERANCE
see Food Allergies, Milk

Lethargy

Most children go through bouts of lethargy and this is partly caused by the huge amount of growth that children have to do. There really are 'growth spurts' which occur after periods when they don't seem to grow a lot.

If your child seems unduly lethargic for more than the odd day, or without an obvious cause – such as insomnia, lack of sleep, anxiety, growth spurt, boredom or having done a lot of physical or other tiring activity – it is worth getting him or her checked out by your doctor. Problems such as anaemia or other illnesses can cause fatigue, as can any illness lasting more than a few days. Some food allergies can also be the culprit.

A poor diet and lifestyle can certainly make matters worse and a good one can help. Try the tips below for a few weeks and you may see a real difference in your child – though you may also be wise to see your doctor.

Tips to help beat child fatigue

→ Encourage regular daily exercise in the fresh air – this can produce better results than going to bed, by oxygenating the system and providing a 'lift'.

→ A generally healthy diet, containing enough of all the vitamins and minerals, and sufficient protein, complex carbohydrate and fat should help avoid chronic fatigue and lethargy.

→ Discourage too many highly refined carbohydrates (such as white bread, biscuits, cakes, sweets) in the diet, particularly during the day. Eaten alone, they can also cause low blood sugar levels, which can lead to feelings of tiredness.

→ Offer regular nutritious meals. The ideal lunch is one that contains good amounts of lean protein with a little unrefined carb, a little fat and plenty of fresh fruit/salad/vegetables. Save high-carb meals for the evening, when the soporific effect may be beneficial and aid sleep. Even then, unrefined carbs will provide higher levels of beneficial vitamins and minerals than refined carbs.

→ Sometimes vegetarian or vegan children, or those who are 'selective eating', may not be getting sufficient iron or B vitamins in the diet, a lack of both of which can cause fatigue.

→ Long periods in front of the TV or computer, combined with lack of circulating air in the room can contribute to fatigue.

See also: Anaemia p135, Anxiety p135, Carbohydrates p144, Food Allergies p162, Insomnia p180.

Meat

Meat is the major source of 'first-class' protein in most Western children's diets. This means that it contains all the essential amino acids (the 'building blocks' of complete protein) that we need. Dairy produce contains complete protein, but most plant sources of protein – e.g. most pulses, and the protein in grains, nuts and seeds – only contain a proportion of these eight amino acids and so vegetarians need to 'mix and match' their protein sources to get all eight necessary for growth, repair and health.

Meat is also a good source of B vitamins (important for growth, nervous system, digestion and usage of food, and body maintenance) and minerals, especially iron and zinc as well as selenium.

Many people feel that meat is not 'healthy' as it contains high levels of fat and saturated fat. If you choose lean cuts, however, beef, pork and even lamb can be low or moderate in both. If buying beefburgers or sausages for your children, go for those labelled 'extra-quality' or 'extra-lean' and grill rather than fry. It is well worth paying extra for premium sausages. The fat in fattier cuts of meat can be reduced by sensible cooking – such as grilling until the fat runs off, or casseroling then cooling and removing the fat from the surface. You can also buy cooks' brushes, which soak up surface liquid fat.

Liver and all other offal, such as kidneys, is very high in a range of vitamins and minerals and is a good source of protein. Kidneys are leaner than liver. However, offal is high in cholesterol and so anyone following a low-cholesterol diet should avoid it. Liver is very high in vitamin A. Large amounts of this vitamin are toxic and can cause birth defects in children, so liver should be avoided during pregnancy and small children should only be given very tiny amounts.

See also: Fats and Oils p157, Food Poisoning p166, Food Safety p167, Poultry and Game p198, Protein p199.

Microwaves

These work by generating electromagnetic energy (microwaves) via a magnetron inside the oven. The microwaves agitate the water molecules in food (all food contains a high percentage of water) and this vibration causes the food to heat up and cook. There has been some speculation over the years that using microwave ovens may cause health problems but, as yet, there is no proof of this. Some experts feel that microwave cooking is healthier than other methods, as more of the water-soluble vitamins B and C may be retained, and foods such as fish or chicken can be cooked without any added fat.

Microwave cooking tends not to be practical for family meals, as it isn't ideal for cooking lots of food at a time. However, if you do use the microwave to reheat food or cook for your children, care should be taken to heat foods right through until piping hot, especially if a food has been defrosted, to prevent food poisoning.

It is best not to heat infant's formula milk in the microwave as it is very easy to overheat – use a jug of warm water instead.

Microwave safety guidelines

→ Follow microwave manufacturers' instructions.
→ Follow instructions on food packaging.
→ Use the right microwave oven equipment (e.g. containers). Anything with metal in it or on it is not suitable – use glass, paper or microwaveable plastics.
→ Defrost food thoroughly before cooking, or according to food packaging instructions.
→ Cook thick pieces of food for longer than thin pieces. Place thick pieces towards the outside of a dish or plate, thin ones in the centre.
→ Stir food during the cooking process to avoid hot and cold spots.
→ Ensure food is piping hot throughout, then let food stand for a few minutes before eating.
→ Keep the oven clean.

Milk

Milk is a good source of calcium – in fact, it is the main source of calcium in many Western children's diets. It also contains some B vitamins, is one of the few major sources of iodine and is a reasonable source of protein. Whole (or full-fat) milk is also a good source of the fat-soluble vitamin A. The proportion of saturates in milk fat is quite high, but if you want to watch your child's overall fat intake, semi-skimmed milk is a good compromise as 100ml contains just over 1.7g fat, compared to whole milk, which contains 3.9g fat.

→ **Under the age of 6 months** – cows' milk shouldn't be given to children at all.

→ **Until aged 1** – a formula milk should be given if not breast-feeding, although from 6 to 12 months small amounts of milk can be given within foods (e.g. custard, cheese sauce). Cows' milk shouldn't be offered as a drink under the age of 1; neither should ordinary unmodified goats' or other types of milk.

→ **Under the age of 2** – whole cows' milk should be given rather than reduced-fat milk, which has less of the fat-soluble vitamins.

→ **Over the age of 2** – semi-skimmed milk can be given, while skimmed milk may be given to children over 5 who are overweight.

Cows'-milk protein (CMP) allergy

A small proportion of young children (about 2% of infants) are allergic to cows'-milk protein (CMP) though this allergy is often outgrown by the age of 3 to 5. CMP allergy symptoms may include sickness, diarrhoea, eczema, wheezing, coughing and a runny nose. Symptoms usually occur within a week to a month of first exposure to cows'-milk formula. Children with CMP allergy need to avoid all cows'-milk protein and products containing it or derivatives (see below). Infants usually take a casein or whey hydrolysate milk formula instead – often the best option as many children with CMP are also allergic to soya formula and may also have a reaction to modified goats'- or sheep's-milk proteins.

CMP – reading the labels

Some products that contain CMP aren't immediately apparent. Obviously all cows' milk needs to be excluded from the diet, as well as products made from cows' milk, which contain protein – e.g. butter, cheese, yoghurt. Less obvious sources are those containing, or that may contain, casein or whey (see below). Look out for these terms on labels: caseinate, caseinate salts, sodium caseinate, hydrolysed whey, whey protein, whey sugar, whey syrup.

If you suspect your child has CMP allergy, you should see your doctor, who should refer you to a dietitian for advice and a full list of foods free of cows'-milk protein.

Foods with hidden CMP protein

→ Soya cheese, vegetarian cheese
→ Margarine and low-fat spreads
→ Some breads
→ Biscuits and rusks
→ Sausages
→ Non-milk-fat ice cream
→ Muesli and other breakfast cereals
→ Fish fingers and fish in batter
→ ...and possibly many other products

Lactose intolerance

This is an allergy to the milk sugars (lactose) rather than the protein, and is a result of the absence of the lactase enzyme, which digests lactose. This causes bloating, stomach ache and other symptoms, and is more common in those of Asian, Indian, Afro-Caribbean and middle Eastern origin, who traditionally did not drink cows' milk. It is also more common in older children of these races, affecting only about 5% of children under 4. About 2% of our total population has lactose intolerance.

Avoiding lactose is not easy as it is used widely in the food industry and may even be present in crisps and sausages. Ironically, several dairy products are not lactose-rich. Hard cheeses contain very little and bio yoghurt may also be tolerated because the fermentation makes them easy to digest. A dietitian can help by suggesting a suitable balanced diet for a lactose-intolerant child, and by providing lists of foods that can be eaten and those that should be avoided. In recent years it has been found that tolerance to lactose can be improved by gradually introducing very tiny amounts of lactose-containing foods, such as cows' milk, into the diet. Some experts find this treatment controversial, but it does seem to work for many. However it should be tried only with the help of a qualified dietitian.

Milk safety

There has been some controversy in recent years about the possibility that our milk is contaminated with antibiotics, pesticide residues, hormones that have been fed to cows to increase their yield (BST) and so on. A bacterium (*Mycobacterium avium* subsp. *paratuberculosis* or MAP) which has been linked to Crohn's Disease has been found in 1.8% of UK pasteurized milk samples. At present there are no official guidelines on these issues, but it's worth noting that low-fat milk contains fewer residues than whole milk because the toxins are stored in the fat. Also, organic milk won't contain BST, the yield hormone, and should be free from pesticide residues. Tests on ultra-heat-treated (UHT) milk have shown that it doesn't contain MAP.

See also: Successful Weaning p10, Allergies and Infants p22, Dairy Produce p150, Food Allergies p162, Food Poisoning p166, Food Safety p167, Pulses p200.

Minerals

Fifteen different minerals are essential in the human diet: calcium, iron, zinc, selenium, magnesium, potassium, iodine, chromium, sodium, phosphorous, copper, fluoride, manganese, cobalt and sulphur. The three main functions of minerals are: in body structure – e.g. calcium is a major component of bone; to control the balance of body fluids; and to regulate all the body functions such as the nervous system and the blood supply. Adequate amounts of minerals are vital for child growth, development and health.

Minerals are present in almost all foods and drinks – even water – but the diet may be deficient in some of those listed, such as iron, selenium and magnesium. The table overleaf lists the minerals that may be in short supply in the diet, with their functions, main sources

MINERALS THAT MAY BE IN SHORT SUPPLY IN THE DIET

Mineral	What it does	Deficiency can cause
Calcium (Ca)	Major constituent of bones and teeth; vital to ensure peak bone mass; helps control muscle/heart function and nervous system.	Rickets, poor bone structure, later osteoporosis; heart problems.
Iron (Fe)	Carries oxygen through the bloodstream; boosts immune system and helps healing.	Anaemia, tiredness, weakness.
Zinc (Zn)	Essential for growth, development and fertility; antioxidant, boosts immune system, helps wound healing.	Retarded growth/sexual development; poor immunity to disease and infection.
Selenium (Se)	Powerful antioxidant protecting against heart disease and cancer; normal growth, fertility and metabolism.	Increased risk of cancer and heart disease, linked with miscarriage and arthritis.
Magnesium (Mg)	Component of bone, works with calcium; releases energy from food and helps nutrient absorption; regulates body functions; helps heart health.	Heart problems, muscle weakness, cramp, appetite loss.
Potassium (K)	Works in conjunction with sodium to regulate body fluid; regulates cell and heart function and blood pressure.	Raised blood pressure; heart problems.
Iodine (I)	Essential for the functioning of the thyroid gland to maintain correct body metabolism and cholesterol levels, regulates oxygen uptake and other vital body functions. During pregnancy, vital for development of the foetal nervous system.	Malfunctions of the thyroid gland, including underactive thyroid which can lead to slowing of metabolic rate, weight gain, coldness, constipation.

Found in	Notes	Recommended daily amounts
All dairy produce especially hard cheeses, milk and yoghurt, dark leafy green vegetables, fortified white bread and fortified cereals.	Absorption helped by vitamin D and essential fatty acids; hindered by phytates in insoluble fibre (e.g. wheat bran) and by oxalates in spinach, rhubarb, beetroot, chocolate.	0–12 months 525mg 1–3 years 350mg 4–6 years 450mg
Red meat especially offal, dark leafy greens, pulses, whole grains, seeds, nuts, dried fruit, fortified cereals.	Absorption is helped by vitamin C in the same meal; hindered by phytates, and oxalates (see Calcium). Excess iron can cause stomach upsets, constipation, kidney damage.	0–3 months 1.7mg 4–6 months 4.3mg 7–12 months 7.8mg 1–3 years 6.9mg 4–6 years 6.1mg
Meat, dairy produce, offal, seeds, shellfish, nuts.	Absorption hindered (as Calcium and Iron). Vegans need to take care to ensure adequate intake. Diet very high in zinc may inhibit copper absorption.	0–6 months 4mg 7 months–3 years 5mg 4–6 years 6.5mg
Nuts, offal, pulses, fish, seeds, meat.	Levels in foods vary greatly depending on the levels in the soil where plant foods grow or where animals graze. Levels in the UK soil may be low. Toxic in excess; upper limit for adults is 450µg a day.	0–3 months 10µg 4–6 months 13µg 7–12 months 10µg 1–3 years 15µg 4–6 years 20µg
Whole grains, nuts, seeds, leafy greens, hard tap water.	Less than half of dietary magnesium is absorbed; absorption may be hindered by a diet rich in sweet foods.	0–3 months 55mg 4–6 months 60mg 7–9 months 75mg 10–12 months 80mg 1–3 years 85mg 4–6 years 120mg
Fruits and vegetables, pulses, nuts.	High sodium (salt) intake increases body's need for potassium. Diuretics and laxatives increase excretion.	0–3 months 800mg 4–6 months 850mg 7–12 months 700mg 1–3 years 800mg 4–6 years 1,100mg
Milk, seafood, seaweed.	Brassicas (e.g. cabbage), sweet potatoes, corn and broad beans inhibit absorption of iodine. Almost half the populations of Europe have been found to be deficient in iodine.	0–3 months 50µg 4–12 months 60µg 1–3 years 70µg 4–6 years 100µg

(not all) and recommended daily amounts for young children – sodium is dealt with in the entry on Salt, page 203.

Minerals are best absorbed as a natural part of food/drink rather than given as supplements – and certain factors hinder or improve their absorption. Most of the minerals are very unlikely to be deficient in the body as they are so widely present and/or are needed in very small quantities. An excess of minerals in the diet isn't wise either, as they can be toxic in large amounts.

There are no UK RDAs (recommended daily amounts) for chromium, but this mineral is important because it helps to promote correct insulin response (diabetes) and blood sugar levels. Meat, offal, eggs, seafood, cheese, whole grains, vegetables and nuts are good sources. A diet high in refined foods and sugars may stimulate the excretion of chromium.

Fluoride is another essential mineral, but again there are no UK RDAs and a deficiency is unlikely. In areas where tap water is fluoridated, high intakes may lead to mottling of the teeth, but fluoridation of water has decreased tooth decay by about 50%.

See also: Diabetes p151, Salt p203.

Muscle development

In order to build optimum lean tissue (muscle) in their bodies, children need a diet that contains adequate protein, minerals – including magnesium – and adequate calories. If enough calories aren't provided

for the child's energy needs, the body will use its stored glycogen (glucose stores), then its stored body fat and then its lean tissue to produce energy. Children also need to take adequate exercise in order to convert dietary protein into muscle.

Nutrients

'Nutrient' is the term used to describe the various components of what we eat and drink that will make a contribution to our nutritional intake. These nutrients are the macronutrients – carbohydrate, fat and protein, which provide the calorie content of our diets; and the micronutrients – the vitamins, minerals, and other compounds that the body needs in small amounts. Dietary fibre isn't a nutrient as such, but is necessary for body function and, of course, we also need water.

See also: Minerals p185, Vitamins p213.

Nuts

Nuts are high in fat, but most varieties are fairly low in saturated fat and high in mono-unsaturates, with the exception of walnuts, which are high in polyunsaturates and contain good amounts of the omega-3 fats as alpha-linolenic acid. In other words, they contain the 'healthy' fats. The exception is the coconut, which is very high in a saturated fat called lauric acid and other saturates.

Nuts are also a good source of protein and fibre, and they provide valuable vitamins and minerals. Almonds, hazelnuts and pecans are some of the best food sources of antioxidant vitamin E, and almonds, cashews, hazelnuts and walnuts contain good amounts of folate. Almonds, in particular, but also Brazils, hazelnuts and walnuts are good sources of calcium. Iron and zinc are present in good amounts in most nuts, but cashews and pecans are particularly high in zinc. Brazils are unique amongst nuts in their very high content of the antioxidant mineral selenium.

Walnuts are a particularly good source of the phytochemical ellagic acid, also found in many fruits. Nuts, eaten on a regular basis, may help to protect against heart disease and some cancers, because of their high antioxidant content. And a diet high in nuts has been shown to significantly reduce LDL cholesterol in the blood.

Nuts are a healthier alternative snack to crisps or sweets for school-age children, but care must be taken to ensure that they are not accessible to children with a nut allergy. For this reason it is considered unwise to pack them in lunch-boxes. Note that nuts should be bought unbroken and stored in a cool dark place to retain their nutrients.

Nut allergies and choking: Nuts shouldn't be given to small children, as they can easily choke on them. Avoid giving children whole nuts until the age of 5, although nut butters can be eaten earlier. Peanut allergy is quite common in children, though some children are allergic to other nuts. Supermarkets and food manufacturers should be able to supply a list of their products which definitely don't contain nuts. The following foods are likely to contain nuts, but a high number of processed foods will have a 'may contain nuts/nut traces' on the label as a precaution.

Foods that may contain nuts:

→ Chocolates   → Sweets   → Toffee

→ Biscuits   → Cakes   → Desserts

→ Baked goods

→ ...any foods produced in a factory that also makes foods containing nuts

See also: Allergies and Infants p22, Peanuts and Food Allergies p56, Antioxidants p135, Essential Fatty Acids p156, Fats and Oils p157, Food Allergies p162, Peanuts p195, Phytochemicals p195, Seeds p204, Contacts p219.

Obesity/overweight

Overweight and obesity among children are ever-increasing problems in this country. Advice for different age groups is given in the first part of the book. Here we look at general strategies for preventing or, as necessary, reversing overweight in children.

What causes obesity?: Weight balance is achieved by matching the amount of energy (kilocalories/joules) that a person consumes in the form of food and drink, with the amount of energy that he or she expends (burns up) in the process of living and, in the case of children, growing and developing. If a child takes in more energy than he or she expends in living, then the surplus calories will be stored as body fat. The more out of kilter the energy balance is, and the more body fat is stored, the more the child becomes overweight and then obese.

Why does it matter?: Children, quite naturally, come in all different shapes and sizes, and there is much variation in what is classed as 'normal weight'. A skinny child and a slightly plump child can both be healthy. If a child is classed as clinically overweight, however, this gives him or her an increased risk of becoming obese in the years ahead, and both clinical overweight and obesity are linked with a variety of health problems – not just when the child reaches adulthood, but often sooner.

Experts believe that childhood obesity is a main cause of increasing incidence of signs of heart disease and diabetes in children. And an overweight child has a much greater chance of becoming an overweight adult, which is linked with not only heart disease and diabetes, but also with some cancers, arthritis, stroke and several other serious health problems.

Is your child overweight?

You can get a good indication as to whether or not your child is a reasonable bodyweight by working out his or her Body Mass Index (BMI) and checking the result against the table.

Body mass index (BMI)

The following instructions will enable you to calculate your child's BMI:
→ Write down your child's height in metres.
→ Square this result (multiply the figure by itself, e.g. 1.25m x 1.25m) using a calculator.
→ Write down your child's weight in kg.
→ Now divide the weight in kg by the height in metres squared. The result is your child's BMI (body mass index).
→ Finally check off your child's BMI against the ages listed in the table. If the BMI is more than that listed, your child is overweight.

BODY MASS INDEX (BMI)
Your child is overweight if he/she is:

Age, years	Boys, BMI over	Girls, BMI over
2	18.4	18
3	17.9	17.6
4	17.6	17.3
5	17.4	17.1
6	17.6	17.3
7	17.9	17.8

So how can overweight be prevented?: There are two ways to keep a child from gaining excess weight, which should complement each other. The first is to make sure that he or she is active and takes enough regular exercise. This burns calories, speeds up their metabolic rate, builds lean tissue (muscle) – which is more metabolically active than other body tissue – and also helps keep the child fit and healthy.

Lack of exercise is certainly a factor in the increase in childhood obesity. Watching television, time at the computer, lack of organized sport at school, transport to school rather than walking or cycling – all combine to give our children a sedentary lifestyle. This means that they need fewer calories in day-to-day living than they used to, say, 50 years ago. But they are not taking in fewer calories.

So the second way to prevent overweight in children is to match their calorie intake to their calorie needs. The Eating Plans for the different age groups (on pages 26–31, 58–66 and 119–121) are a good starting point. They offer a balance of carbohydrates, fat and protein, and are low on sugar and other foods that are high in calories but low in nutrients.

Preventing a child becoming overweight

The following tips will help to ensure that your child has a healthy well-balanced diet without excessive calories:

→ Restrict sugary sweets, drinks and snacks, such as packet cakes and biscuits.

→ Restrict snacks that are high in fat, especially highly processed snacks, such as crisps. Fresh fruit is the best between-meal snack.

→ Offer fruit-based desserts rather than high-fat/high-sugar ready-made desserts.

→ Try to get your child to drink bottled water or semi-skimmed milk rather than high-sugar drinks or full-fat milkshakes – this can save hundreds of calories.

→ Cook with less fat at home. This will help the whole family reduce their fat intake.

→ Avoid burger bars and fish 'n' chip shops. Much fast food is very high in fat and calories.

→ Try to match portion sizes to your child's appetite and needs. It is better for a child to ask for more if still hungry at the end of a meal rather than have a plate piled high – children tend to eat what is on their plate, even if full.

And if your child is already overweight...

Most experts feel that if a child is still growing in height, the best course of action is to try to maintain the current weight and, as the child grows taller, he or she will literally grow into their correct weight. Exercising some control over their calorie intake is still important, to make sure they doesn't put on more weight.

If your child is obese, visit your doctor who will refer you to a dietitian to obtain a suitable eating plan, as it is unlikely that your child will slim down naturally without intervention.

The hungry overweight child: If an overweight child has his or her calorie intake reduced too drastically or too suddenly, he or she will probably feel both hungry and resentful.

Tips to stop the overweight child feeling hungry:

→ Choose foods that are low on the Glycaemic Index (see overleaf) as snacks for your child. This is an index used by dietitians to measure how long carbohydrate foods take to be absorbed into the bloodstream once they are eaten. A food that takes a short time (e.g. glucose, sugar) has a high GI rating, while one that takes a long time (e.g. pulses, apple) has a low GI rating.

The Glycaemic Index measures only carbohydrate foods, but both fat and protein take a long time to be absorbed into the bloodstream and, when eaten with a high-GI food, have the effect of lowering its GI rating. Low-GI foods will help keep hunger at bay, medium low- or medium-GI foods are fairly good at doing so, but high-GI foods – unless eaten as part of a meal containing fat, protein and/or low-GI carbs – will soon have the child feeling hungry again.

→ Feed little and often.

→ Encourage the child to eat slowly and chew well.

→ Provide plenty of high-fibre foods, which often take longer to eat than highly refined foods (compare eating an apple with having a glass of apple juice). Most high-fibre foods also take longer to be digested.

→ Give your child plenty of low-calorie drinks (e.g. water) with a meal; this also helps a feeling of fullness.

The Glycaemic Index

Low-GI foods: All pulses (e.g. baked beans, butter beans, chickpeas) and foods made from them (e.g. hummus); wholewheat pasta; whole-rye grain; barley; apples, peaches, cherries, grapefruit, plums, oranges, pears, dried apricots; most green vegetables, avocados, onions, peppers, tomatoes, yoghurt, milk, nuts.

Medium-low- or medium-GI foods: Sweetcorn, peas, root vegetables except mashed and baked potatoes; carrots; white pasta, oats, popcorn, noodles; dark rye bread; pitta; bulghar wheat; white and brown basmati rice; slightly underripe bananas, grapes, dates, figs, kiwi fruit.

High-GI foods: Glucose, sugar, honey, sweets, lollies, pineapple, raisins, melon, ripe bananas; baked or mashed potatoes; non-basmati brown and white rice; wholemeal and white bread; couscous; cornflakes and similar cereals.

The Traffic Light System

A less formal way to help an overweight child over 5 to eat fewer calories is the 'traffic light' system. This categorizes foods into either Red for 'stop', Amber for 'proceed with caution' or Green for 'go'.

This way neither you nor the child needs to be worried about calorie-counting and, as long as you give him or her plenty of foods from the Green section, they needn't have a meagre plateful. As you look through the list, the categories may seem obvious, but if you stick to the rules the system really will help you control your child's weight.

Green for Go – eat as much as you like:

→ Fruit – fresh, frozen, or canned in water or natural juice
→ Vegetables – fresh, frozen or canned in water including plainly cooked potatoes
→ Fresh salad items
→ Whole grains; wholewheat pasta; pulses
→ Wholegrain breads, good-quality white bread and breakfast cereals
→ Dried apricots and prunes
→ Fish and shellfish
→ Lean poultry and lean red meat
→ Natural yoghurt and fromage frais; skimmed or semi-skimmed milk, low- or medium-fat cheeses
→ Quorn, tofu

Amber for Proceed with Caution – eat in moderate portions or occasionally:

→ Refined grain products (e.g. breakfast cereal)
→ Eggs, full-fat cheese, whole milk
→ Olive oil, groundnut oil, rapeseed oil
→ Nuts and seeds
→ Low-fat spread, reduced-fat salad dressings
→ Fruit juice
→ Oven chips, roast potatoes, mashed potato
→ Low-fat custard, low-fat rice pudding

Red for Stop and Think – avoid or eat in very tiny amounts or very occasionally:

→ Sweets
→ Cakes, biscuits, pastry, puddings
→ Butter, lard, margarine, cream
→ Crisps, salted nuts, other salted snacks
→ Deep-fried foods, battered foods
→ Fatty cuts of meat
→ Sugary squashes and soft fizzy drinks
→ Takeaways, such as pizzas, fish and chips

Low-fat foods – any use?

In the shops you see lots of products labelled 'reduced-fat' 'low-fat' or 'fat-free', and some of these are foods normally very high in fat. Is it worth buying these for your child?

Research suggests that overall reduced-fat products don't actually help anyone to lose weight. This may be because, although the fat is reduced, the product may not be much lower in calories, as there may be extra sugar or other ingredients added. It may also be because when people buy reduced-fat reduced-calorie products they tend to eat more of them, or more of other foods instead.

Often, the taste/texture/satisfaction quotient of low-fat foods doesn't compare to the original. However, low-fat spreads and lower-fat salad dressings can save a lot of unnecessary fat, and low-fat custard and rice puddings are both useful for quick puddings.

See also: Food Additives p159, Hunger p179.

Onions

Onions, leeks and garlic are all from the same family and all contain phytochemicals called allylic sulphides, which convert to allicin in the body and help to protect against heart disease, some cancers and infections such as colds and coughs. The members of the onion family are also all very low in fat. Children often prefer the milder red onions, which are a good source of the phytochemical quercetin – frying them in oil helps to preserve this compound. Garlic is a particularly powerful antioxidant, rating third on the ORAC scale (Oxygen Radical Absorbance Capacity). Many children find the bulb too pungent, but if it is crushed and used in casseroles, stews, soups, mince dishes and so on, the taste becomes mild. New-season's garlic is also milder than over-wintered garlic, and the plant chemicals are more potent when the garlic is fresh.

Organic food

Organic produce is difficult to discuss as an entity, because it embraces so many different types of food, from many countries, produced in different growing conditions, with varying degrees of care. Organic standards vary from country to country and a lot of the organic food that we eat in the UK is imported.

Because proper organic food is grown in a more traditional way, it often tastes better than mass-produced food. Usually, the best-tasting organic food is that which is sourced locally. There seems to be much less taste difference in imported organic produce and processed organic foods. So if you have a choice, try to buy local organic produce.

Cost is a major consideration for most parents and organic foods range from being between 20% and 70% more expensive than their non-organic equivalents. So, it probably makes sense to buy organic when it really might make the most significant difference to your child's diet.

Nutritional and health benefits

Vitamins and minerals: Several trials have shown that fresh organic produce may contain higher levels of some vitamins and minerals than equivalent non-organic food. This could be because organic food may be given longer to reach maturity or may be grown with more care on non-impoverished soil.

However, if organic fruit and vegetables are not stored well, or stored too long, they may also lose vital nutrients, like vitamins B and C, before you can eat them. This is why it's important to buy your fresh produce, whether organic or not, from a shop where it is kept in cool, non-bright conditions and turnover is high. As an example, avoid box schemes where your box of produce arrives after a day in a hot van looking decidedly wilted and sad.

It has also been shown that organically reared meat and poultry has a much lower water content than factory-farmed meat. This will mean that the meat should cook better, cut better and contain more nutrients than watery mass-market meats. B vitamins in meat will also leach away in the water that comes out of such meat when it is cooked.

Fat content: Ironically, many organic meats contain higher levels of fat, because traditional rearing methods are more likely to result in fattier animals. If you choose the lower-fat ways to cook most of the time, this shouldn't be a problem. Conversely, factory-farmed salmon is fattier than wild salmon because of its unnatural diet and lack of exercise.

Health benefits: The main reason why most people buy organic is to avoid consuming the residues (e.g. pesticides, herbicides, fertilizers in plant foods, colourings and antibiotics in eggs) that may be present in mass-produced foods. These residues, if ingested in quantity, could have potentially serious side-effects over the years. In the UK, very few chemicals are allowed in organic farming, while in non-organic farming there is a list of over 300 that are permitted. Use of antibiotics, growth hormones and medicines is strictly limited, as is the use of non-organic feed to farm animals. Also, foods containing GM ingredients will not be certified as organic in the UK.

Our non-organic food is frequently tested for what are considered safe levels of residues. However, as we are being encouraged to eat more fruit and vegetables, the cumulative intake may be higher than is wise. So, if you can afford to buy just some organic food, I suggest you invest in organic fruits, salads and vegetables, particularly those that won't be peeled. Peeling removes much of the residues, but also takes away the nutrients that are concentrated in, or just under, the skin in many fruits and vegetables. Lettuces, leafy greens and carrots tend to retain more residues than other vegetables, so opt for organic. Buy organic citrus fruits if you are going to use the peel (e.g. in marmalade or desserts) and if your children eat a lot of dried fruit, buy organic, because it doesn't contain the sulphur preservatives that are linked with allergy in some children.

Organic flour and bread are good choices, but remember that organic bread is unlikely to keep as long as standard manufactured bread. As far as processed food is concerned, just because a pack says the contents are organic, it doesn't necessarily mean that the food inside is especially good, or tasty.

See also: Food Additives p159, Food Standards p170, Health Foods p178, Whole Foods p218.

Peanuts

Peanuts are ground nuts rather than tree nuts, and their oil is called groundnut oil. Peanuts contain a wide range of vitamins and minerals and they are particularly rich in potassium and magnesium. Like most nuts, they are very high in calories because of their high fat content, and so are best eaten in small portions, unless the child is underweight.

Peanuts are a good source of resveratrol, a phytochemical that helps protect against heart disease and some cancers. Peanuts can be added to stir-fries, chopped and added to veggy burgers, or sprinkled over salads. Good-quality peanut butter has a similar nutrient and resveratrol profile to peanuts.

Don't give peanuts to children under 5 in case they have an undiagnosed peanut allergy. Whole nuts of any kind shouldn't be given to those under 5 because of the risk of choking.

Peanut allergy isn't uncommon in very young children and it can be very serious, even life-threatening. Groundnut oil can produce an allergic reaction in children with a severe peanut allergy. Peanuts or peanut traces may be present in many commercial foods, including cakes, chocolate, biscuits, desserts and all processed foods made in factories which also handle peanuts, as contamination is a possibility. Supermarkets and food manufacturers should be able to provide you with a list of foods that definitely do not contain nuts or peanuts.

See also: Peanuts and Food Allergies p56, Food Allergies p162, Minerals p185, Nuts p188, Phytochemicals p195.

Peppers

Sweet peppers are a very useful vegetable for children as they are sweet and juicy (particularly the red, orange and yellow varieties) and can be used raw or cooked in very many dishes. Once cooked, they become sweeter and the high levels of beta-carotene that the red colours contain are better absorbed if cooked in a little oil. Sweet peppers are also very high in vitamin C. Red peppers contain a particular carotenoid antioxidant called beta-cryptoxanthin, which helps to prevent heart disease.

Phytochemicals

These are a range of beneficial chemicals and compounds found in plant material – fruits, vegetables, grains, pulses, nuts and seeds. Many of them have antioxidant properties and are linked with reduced risk of heart disease, cancers and ill health. They may be even more important in the diet than vitamins and minerals (some of which also have an antioxidant effect), and many experts believe that this is why taking vitamin/mineral supplements is not a substitute for eating whole fruits, etc. Cooking doesn't necessarily destroy phytochemicals, in fact sometimes their absorption can be enhanced through cooking. Carotenoids, in particular, are better absorbed when cooked with oil. The chart on the following pages gives the role of the various phytochemicals and lists those foods that are good sources.

See also: Antioxidants p135.

PHYTOCHEMICALS

FLAVONOLS (PHENOLIC COMPOUNDS)

Phytochemical	Found in	What it does (action)
Anthocyanins	Blueberries, blackberries, blackcurrants, cherries, cranberries, black grapes, strawberries, raspberries, red-tinged leaves.	Antioxidant, anti-inflammatory.
Catechins (flavanols)	Apples, chocolate, cocoa, tea (green/black), pears, wine.	Antioxidant, heart protection.
Flavanones	Citrus fruits, prunes, cashew nuts.	Antioxidant, cholesterol-lowering.
Flavones	Artichokes, celery, lemons, parsley, peppers, olives, oranges.	Antioxidant, anti-cancer.
Quercetin	Apples, citrus fruits, grapes, lettuce (red-tinged), onions, tea.	Anti-cancer, skin-protecting, cataract prevention, anti-hay fever.
Rutin	Citrus fruits.	Antioxidant, heart health.

OTHER PHENOLS

Phytochemical	Found in	What it does (action)
Capsaicin	Chillies, peppers.	Antioxidant, pain killer, anti-inflammatory, cholesterol-lowering.
Coumarins	Citrus fruits, green tea, leafy green vegetables, parsley.	Help to prevent blood clotting, anti- cancer.
Curcumin	Corn, mustard, turmeric.	Antioxidant, anti-inflammatory.
Ellagic acid	Black and red berries, cherries, grapes, pecans, walnuts.	Anti-cancer.
Resveratrol	Red grape juice, red wine.	Antioxidant, heart protection.

CAROTENOIDS

Phytochemical	Found in	What it does (action)
Alpha-carotene	Avocado, carrots, corn, red peppers, squash, tomatoes.	Antioxidant, anti-cancer.
Beta-carotene	Carrots, dark leafy greens, sweet potatoes, red peppers, orange-fleshed squash, cantaloupe melon.	Anti-cancer, immune-booster, eye health, skin health.
Cryptoxanthin	Red, orange and yellow fruits.	Heart health.
Lutein	Dark leafy greens, peas, rhubarb, squash.	Eye health.
Lycopene	Tomatoes, pink grapefruit.	Anti-cancer, anti-heart disease.
Zeaxanthin	Lettuce, spinach, spring greens, sweetcorn.	Eye health.

PHYTO OESTROGENS

Phytochemical	Found in	What it does (action)
Coumestrol	Beansprouts.	Anti-inflammatory.
Isoflavones	Soya and soya products, and other pulses.	Heart health, possible breast cancer risk reduction.
Lignans	Linseed, whole grains, berries.	Possibly anti-breast cancer.

OTHERS

Phytochemical	Found in	What it does (action)
Glucosinolates	Broccoli (sulphoraphanes), cabbage (indoles), cauliflower, kale, Brussels sprouts (sinigrin).	Anti-cancer.
Lentinen	Exotic mushrooms, e.g. shiitake.	Immune-boosting, anti-cancer.
Phytosterols	Soya beans, nuts, seeds, whole grains.	LDL cholesterol-lowering.
Sulphides	Garlic, onions, leeks.	Antioxidant, anti-bacterial, anti-cancer, heart and circulation protection.

Potatoes

Potatoes are a starchy carbohydrate food, which also contains some protein, virtually no fat and a range of vitamins and minerals as well as fibre. They make a useful contribution to most children's vitamin C intake and also provide energy. Roast potatoes and mash can be almost as high in fat as chips (see below), so if you need to watch the family's fat intake go easy with the butter in your mash, and try dry-roasting the potatoes by just brushing scrubbed potato chunks with olive oil to bake. Use groundnut oil or light olive oil for roasting rather than blended vegetable oil or lard.

The skin is a good source of fibre and the flesh just under the skin contains much of the vitamin C, so try to use potatoes well scrubbed but unpeeled. New potatoes contain most vitamin C – indeed, potatoes that have been overwintered, then stored in a warm spot may contain very little. Don't peel potatoes and then leave them soaking, as vitamin C will leach out. Cooking potatoes with a little oil or baking them loses less vitamin C than boiling. Avoid green potato, as it contains toxins.

Chips

Deep-fried chips are the least healthy way to eat potatoes because they are high in calories, fat and/or saturated fat, and lately they have been linked with high levels of acrylamide, a potential carcinogen. If a child eats a lot of chips it may well contribute to overweight.

If you deep-fry your own chips, choose a good-quality oil, such as groundnut or rapeseed oil and replace it regularly. Cook chips only once – don't refry them as they will soak up yet more fat – and serve them straight away to retain the vitamin C. The same guidelines apply to ready-cut chips for frying.

For a healthier option, make your own oven chips (see Potato Wedges, page 81). Commercial oven chips come with the fat impregnated in the chip, so that all you have to do is bake them. They do contain a little less fat than standard fried chips. Go for the larger ones and straight-cuts, which will have less total fat than small ones or crinkle cuts.

Take-away chips can be very unhealthy, especially large fish-shop portions, which have been cooked in hard or blended vegetable oils. Most burger chains now use healthier cooking fats, but they are generally thinly cut so they absorb a lot of oil.

See also: Carbohydrates p144, Fats and Oils p157, Fried Food p172, Obesity p189.

Poultry and game

The lean meat from all poultry and game (dark meat or light) is reasonably low in fat. But, if you eat chicken with its skin, or a duck portion with the fat layer intact, then the dish can be as high, or higher, in fat than red meat.

Poultry and game is an excellent source of protein and a good source of B vitamins and many minerals. Poor-quality poultry is often laced with a great deal of added water and may even contain other meats, e.g. pork, so try to buy good-quality meat.

Other game meats, such as venison and pheasant, have a similar vitamin and mineral content, although venison is very low in fat, while pheasant is higher in fat than chicken.

Salmonella may be present in poultry. It is therefore essential to cook poultry all the way through, leaving no pink flesh, to kill the salmonella bug and protect the family against food poisoning.

See also: Food Poisoning p166, Meat p182, Protein p199, Ready Meals p202.

Processed foods

All food is processed in one form or another before you eat it – even cutting a lettuce from the garden could be described as processing it. However, what we usually mean by processed food is that which looks, or is, substantially different from its original ingredient(s) and this has evolved into a huge industry. There are several reasons for food processing:

→ To preserve food in a fit state to eat.
→ To add value, interest and/or palatability.
→ To use up by-products: e.g. the skimmed-off cream from whole milk in desserts, etc.

Although food processing has given us more variety, interest and convenience in the form of long-life items, it has drawbacks. Some processed foods are a nutritious part of a child's diet – canned tomatoes, tomato purée, tomato passata, pulses, fish canned in water and frozen foods, for example.

However, many processed foods are high in fat, saturates, trans fats, salt and/or sugar, and food additives. Canned vegetables and fruits may contain less vitamin C and B than fresh or frozen, and the vital plant chemicals may be missing from many products. At its worst, food processing strips the original food of many important nutrients and then adds a list of ingredients that are unhealthy and/or unnecessary to health, and/or artificial.

If you rely on a lot of cans, packs, jars and so on to feed your children, buy the best quality you can afford, read the labels and supplement them with plenty of fresh fruit, salads and vegetables. And try the recipes in this book – most of them are quick and easy.

See also: Drinks p153, Food Additives p159, Ready Meals p202, Salt p203, Sugar and Sweeteners p205.

Protein

Protein is needed in all children's diets to provide the 'building blocks' for body maintenance, repair and growth. Proteins are essential constituents of all cells; they also regulate body processes and provide structure. The formation of lean tissue (muscle and other non-fat and non-bone structures) is dependent upon regular adequate protein in the diet. While surplus protein can be converted into energy, the body cannot convert carbohydrate or fat into protein.

Proteins in foods are formed from chains of amino acids and there are eight essential amino acids that the body must get from its food (plus a ninth, which is important in infancy but not needed afterwards). Some foods, mainly animal sources of protein, contain all eight of these amino acids and these are sometimes called 'complete proteins'. While others, mainly pulses and grains, contain only a few and are sometimes called 'incomplete proteins'; soya beans do contain all eight essential amino acids and are unique amongst pulses in this respect.

As the amino acids work best when eaten together, children who eat little animal protein foods (e.g. vegetarians or vegans) can increase the quality of the plant protein foods by combining them within meals so that they form a 'complete protein'.

Some examples of this are:
→ Combine a grain food with a pulse food: e.g., baked beans on toast; hummus and pitta bread; rice and beans.
→ Combine a pulse with nuts/seeds: e.g., lentils and nuts in a carrot salad; sesame seeds with chickpeas in tahini.
→ An incomplete protein with a complete protein: e.g., meat-free chilli con carne made from red kidney beans topped with a little grated cheese; yoghurt with nuts and seeds.

Good sources of protein
Very good sources:
→ **Lean meat, poultry and game**
→ **Fish and shellfish**
→ **Eggs**
→ **Cheese**
→ **Quorn (mycoprotein)**
→ **Peanuts** (only for non-allergic over 5's)
Good sources:
→ **Milk, yoghurt and fromage frais**
→ **Most nuts and seeds**
→ **Pulses, especially soya and tofu**
Very good sources:
→ **Whole grains**
→ **Potatoes**

Choose low-fat protein foods at least some of the time to help moderate your child's total fat and saturated fat intake.

A very high protein intake (especially of animal protein) is linked with a high fat intake as most sources of protein in children's diets are also potentially high in fat – especially dairy produce and meat. So don't be tempted to think that if adequate protein is vital, twice as much is even better – it isn't.

See also: Dairy Produce p150, Eggs p156, Fish p159, Meat p182, Nuts p188, Pulses (below), Seeds p204.

Pulses
Pulses are an extremely useful food group for all the family – they are high in both protein and carbohydrate, low or very low in fat and saturates, and high in fibre. Many are also good sources of some vitamins and excellent sources of minerals. They are low on the Glycaemic Index (see page 192) and so are useful for regulating blood sugar levels and preventing between-meal hunger. They are also inexpensive. Canned pulses are very convenient and have a similar nutritional profile to cooked dried beans, although potassium may be lower, and sodium content much higher if pulses canned in brine are used – so buy them canned in water.

Most pulses are a source of isoflavones and other phytochemical compounds of the phyto-oestrogen family. Soya beans are the richest source of these plant oestrogens.

Cooking tips for pulses
→ If using dried beans, always soak them overnight or as recommended on the packet, change the soaking water before cooking and boil rapidly for 10 minutes or as instructed on

the pack. This will destroy substances in the beans called lectins, which can cause food poisoning-like symptoms if they are eaten undercooked. Lentils don't need fast boiling.

→ Use whole cooked pulses to replace some of the meat in casseroles, curries, pies, meat sauces and stews.

→ Use pulses in vegetable soups to increase the mineral, fibre and calorie content – purée the soup for a fine, smooth texture.

→ Cooked pulses can be added to winter salads – e.g. lentils with grated carrot, chickpeas with red peppers.

→ Cooked pulses can be puréed with a little olive oil and lemon juice to make a dip, spread or pâté.

→ Tofu (beancurd) is a smooth lean protein made from soya beans, which is very useful for vegans in stir-fries, soups, casseroles, etc. Tofu comes in a variety of forms – e.g. silken, smoked.

→ TVP (textured vegetable protein), which is soya-based, can be used as a meat replacement for chunks of meat or minced meat in a dish.

Soya beans

Soya beans are similar to the other pulses in most respects – however they do have a few major differences:

→ They are a 'complete protein' – unlike most plant foods and pulses, they contain all eight essential amino acids that can form complete protein, so they are especially important for vegans and vegetarians.

→ They are relatively high in fat. Soya beans contain a high percentage of fats compared with other pulses, including significant amounts of omega-3 oils.

→ They are very high in isoflavones and other compounds of the phyto-oestrogen family. One isoflavone, called genistein, has been shown to lower LDL blood cholesterol. Other isoflavones in soya may help to maintain bone density and prevent osteoporosis, and may even provide protection against some forms of cancer.

There is much speculation, and research is currently in progress, about possible health concerns related to the high plant oestrogen content of soya. In particular, soya intake during pregnancy, while breast-feeding and in infancy may increase the risk of male fertility problems later in life for the child. Much of the research to date seems to indicate that this may be the case.

See also: Allergies and Infants p22, Essential Fatty Acids p156, Milk p184, Obesity p189, Phytochemicals p195, Protein p199.

Quorn

Quorn is a 'man-made' high-protein food based on 'mycoprotein', which is a relative of the mushroom family. Quorn contains no animal or dairy ingredients and it is moderately low in fat (31% of its total calories are fat calories) and saturates. Quorn doesn't contain a wealth of vitamins and it has a relatively high sodium content, but otherwise this product makes a good substitute for meat. Recent research, however, has shown that it can cause asthma in susceptible individuals.

Ready meals

Ready meals – mass-produced, pre-cooked meals that only require reheating – vary tremendously in their nutrient profile and while some are perfectly acceptable as an occasional meal for your child, others are not good. A significant number contain very little in the way of vegetables and few contain more than a trace of vitamin C. Fibre content is often low as manufacturers tend not to use whole grains for their carbohydrate element. Salt content can be high, some ready meals have an unacceptably high level of fat and many have long lists of food additives.

Improve the nutritional status of ready meals by adding some vegetables or a salad, or at least follow the meal with some fruit. Bear in mind that you get what you pay for, and that chilled meals are likely to be nicer and better nutritionally than frozen ones.

See also: Food Additives p159, Salt p203.

Root vegetables

People often think of root vegetables as high in starchy carbohydrate and little else – in fact, only some roots, such as artichoke, parsnip, sweet potato and yams are high or moderately high in starch. Others, such as carrots, beetroot and swede, are moderately high in carbohydrate, but much of this is in the form of sugars. Another misconception is that root vegetables are high in calories, but mostly they are not. Roots are all low in fat with only a trace of saturates, and some (especially parsnips, which are also the best

source of fibre) contain good amounts of vitamins and minerals. Several are good sources of vitamin C, notably parsnips, swede and sweet potato. Beetroot are one of the best sources of folate, but not if they are pickled.

Orange-fleshed sweet potatoes are an excellent source of carotenoids and vitamins. Another benefit compared with ordinary potatoes is that sweet potatoes have a much lower rating on the Glycaemic Index (see page 192). Jerusalem artichokes are rich in fructo-oligosaccharides, which help build up 'good' bacteria in the gut – useful for children with digestive problems or constipation.

Ideally, root vegetables should be bought in season to maximize their nutrient content. Most children enjoy at least some of the root vegetables apart from potatoes. Carrots are almost always a favourite and beetroot is deliciously sweet, as long as its not pickled.

Tips for serving children root vegetables
→ Bake beetroot in their skins, then peel and slice for a sweet vegetable; or parboil and then grate into winter salads. Avoid pickling as this destroys their important folate content.
→ Cube a selection of root vegetables, toss them in oil and seasoning, and bake for about 50 minutes, turning halfway – great with the Sunday roast as a change from roast potatoes. Or top with cheese sauce and breadcrumbs and brown under the grill for a winter supper.
→ Thinly slice root vegetables, toss them in olive oil, season, lay on a baking tray and bake, turning halfway through cooking, until they are crisp and golden – a healthier option to commercial crisps.

→ Cut root vegetables into large crudités, toss in olive oil and bake until golden, then serve with a cheese or tomato dip.

→ Peel, cube and steam root vegetables until tender, then mash with equal parts potato for a change from basic mash; or mash two different roots together – carrot with parsnip is excellent.

→ Bake sweet potatoes in their skins, or peel, cube and mash them, in the same way as ordinary potatoes – they go particularly well with chicken and beef.

See also: Carrots p145, Phytochemicals p195, Potatoes p198, Vitamins p213.

Salt

Salt consists of 40% sodium and 60% chloride, two minerals which are present in small amounts in virtually all basic foods, including fruit and vegetables. We need a little sodium in our diets – it helps to balance our body fluids and is necessary for the proper functioning of our nerves and muscles – but a little is all we need.

Salt has been used for centuries as a preservative and a flavour enhancer, but it is only in fairly recent years that it has been used in relatively large amounts in food manufacturing. Indeed, experts now estimate that 75% of the salt we consume comes from processed foods, while only 9% is added in cooking at home and 6% added at the table.

Health experts have been worried for some time about our high intake of salt. A 3-year-old child dietary requirement is only 500mg sodium per day, a 6-year-old needs 700mg, while an infant aged 10-12 months requires only 350mg. According to surveys, children are consuming at least twice as much salt as they need.

In 2003 the UK Scientific Committee on Nutrition concluded that there is a direct association between high salt intake and high blood pressure, heart disease and stroke. Other research indicates that a diet high in salt is also linked with increased risk of asthma, osteoporosis, stomach cancer and fluid retention.

To address the problem of high sodium in the diet, guidelines for maximum salt intake have been set. The average daily amount of salt should be less than 1g for a baby up to 6 months; 1g for a 7-12-month infant; 2g for a child aged 1-3; and 3g for a child aged 4-6. It is important to remember that 1g salt is equivalent to 400mg sodium.

What are the high sodium (salt) foods?
Many processed foods have a high salt content – and not just the obvious ones, such as crisps and savoury snacks. Breakfast cereals are a big source of dietary salt – cornflakes, for example, are estimated weight for weight to contain more salt than sea water. A lot of bread is high in salt, and so are most baked beans, even though they taste sweet. Takeaways and canned foods are also typically high in salt. Government guidelines suggest that all products with over 500mg sodium (1.25g salt) per 100g product should be considered to be high in salt – and those are guidelines for adults.

Foods or food groups often particularly high in sodium include: cereals, crackers, savoury snacks, canned soups and vegetables in brine; fish canned in brine; stock cubes; bacon, dried packet soups and sauces; cook-in, stir-in or pour-over ready-made sauces; processed cheeses; smoked foods; soya sauce and some other bottled sauces; takeaway chicken nuggets, burgers and pizzas. Butter and margarine can contain quite high levels too – about 75mg sodium for a 10g portion.

How to reduce your child's sodium intake

→ Try not to encourage a taste for salt from the start. Children who are not used to very salty flavours find salty foods almost unpalatable.

→ Research shows that if you reduce salt in the child's diet gradually over several weeks the taste buds alter and previously enjoyed foods seem far too salty.

→ Read food labels to check sodium content (see right).

→ Stop adding salt to cooked vegetables and at the table.

→ Go for low-salt versions of favourite foods – e.g. baked beans, crisps, butter, bacon, ketchup. Every little saving does add up.

→ Keep to low-salt snacks – a significant percentage of children's salt intake is in the form of snacks.

→ If you buy ready meals and soups, opt for fresh chilled ones rather than long-life canned or dried ones, which often contain a lot more sodium.

→ Restrict high-salt preserved and processed meats – e.g. sausages, frankfurters, burgers.

Salt and food labels

→ The nutrition panel may give sodium content per 100g, but bear in mind that this isn't necessarily the same as a portion.

→ More than 500mg of sodium per 100g food is considered 'a lot'.

→ Manufacturers are obliged to list sodium per portion if they make a claim for salt content on the front of the pack. Try to work out how this relates to your child's maximum target intake.

→ Don't confuse sodium and salt. As salt is 40% sodium, 1g (1000mg) sodium equals 2.5g (2500mg) salt. Some manufacturers list salt content, not sodium content.

→ If there is no sodium listed on the nutrition panel, check the ingredients list for sodium – the higher up the list it appears, the more sodium the product will contain.

See also: Ready Meals p202.

Seeds

Seeds can make a good contribution to a child's diet, providing many minerals that are not found in quantity in a wide variety of foods – such as zinc and selenium. Though high in fat, it is mostly polyunsaturated and there are some of the important omega-3s present in most seeds.

Seeds can be used as snacks, on their own or included with nuts, sprinkled on breakfast cereal, chopped fruit or yoghurt, sprinkled into salads or used in homemade breads and bakes. Eating them raw preserves more of the nutrients. Store seeds in a sealed container in the fridge and eat within a few weeks to ensure the polyunsaturated oils don't oxidize.

Linseed (flax seeds) is not widely available but can be bought at health-food shops and has the highest omega-3 content of all seeds. Tahini – sesame seed paste, commonly used in hummus – is a concentrated source of all the goodness of seeds.

Seeds – particularly sesame seeds – may produce an allergic reaction in some children and should also not be given to very small children as there may be a risk of choking.

See also: Allergies and Infants p22, Essential Fatty Acids p156, Food Allergies p162, Pulses p200, Hummus p73.

SOYA
see Pulses

Stomach upset

'I've got tummy ache!' is a cry all parents are likely to hear many times and there can be numerous causes. If a child has persistent stomach ache or accompanying problems, such as fever, vomiting or diarrhoea, for more than a day or two, then see your doctor.

Stomach ache, no other symptoms:
If the child says they have stomach ache but you can find nothing else wrong, the cause could be psychological (doesn't want to go to school that day or is under stress). If this happens several times you may be able to link the problem to a particular issue (e.g. sports at school). The child may not actually be making up the stomach pains as stress can cause physical symptoms.

Otherwise, try to find out whether the child has eaten something that could cause stomach pains. For example, too many apples or under-ripe bananas. Check also that the child isn't constipated.

Stomach ache, other symptoms:
With other symptoms such as a temperature, hot head, drowsiness, vomiting and/or diarrhoea, it could be food poisoning. It could also be food allergy. Any or all of these together could be symptoms of some other illness, in which case see your doctor. With constipation, the stomach ache should go away when the constipation is relieved.

A bloated, tight-looking stomach could simply be too much food in one session, e.g. from a kids' party. Stomach ache with bloating could, again, be food allergy. Bloating and pains can also be caused by too much sodium, which retains fluid in the body, or by too much refined carbohydrate, which has a similar effect.

See also: Carbohydrates p144, Constipation p148, Food Allergies p162, Food Poisoning p166, Salt p203.

Sugar and sweeteners

The calorie content of sugar and the other sweeteners is all, or virtually all, in the form of sugars. Only honey, syrup and treacle have traces of protein. Sugar contains no vitamins, and its mineral content is insignificant. Syrup is similarly low in nutrients. Honey contains traces of some B vitamins and minerals, but not in any appreciable quantity. However, good-quality honey has antiseptic properties. Treacle has minerals, such as calcium, magnesium and iron, and even quite small quantities of treacle contain good amounts.

Fructose, the sugar in fruit has about the same number of calories as ordinary sugar (sucrose) but it is much sweeter, so about half the amount can be used to achieve the same sweetness as sugar. It is also absorbed into the bloodstream less rapidly than sucrose, and may help lower 'bad' LDL cholesterol in the blood. However, it may cause diarrhoea and have other side-effects if used excessively.

A teaspoonful of sugar contains about 20 calories (4 calories per g). Honey contains only around 14 calories a teaspoonful, but is less sweet so more may need to be used.

Sugar consumption and health

On average, over half of the carbohydrate intake of pre-school children is in the form of sugars rather than starches. Two-thirds of these sugars are in the form of non-milk extrinsic sugars (NMES), i.e. from items such as sweets and sugars added in food processing, rather than from milk or from natural foods such as fruits, vegetables, nuts, seeds and grains. It is estimated that nearly 20% of children's total calorie intake is in the form of extrinsic sugars – nearly double the recommended amount of 10% of total diet. The maximum daily sugar intake should be around 30g for a child aged 1-3, and about 40g for a child aged 4-6. About three-quarters of this sugar intake is from processed foods and drinks, rather than sugar added to foods at home. This is a concern because there is plenty of evidence that a high sugar intake is not good for our children.

Sugar and weight While a diet high in natural, starchy complex carbohydrates and intrinsic sugars (found within the structure of the food – e.g. in fruit) is linked with good health and ease of weight maintenance, a diet high in non-milk extrinsic sugars (NMES) is linked with obesity. It is foods such as chocolates, sweets, sugary desserts, cakes and biscuits, which are most likely to be eaten when children are not hungry. Such foods are often also high in fat and low in fibre and are very easy to eat. Simply cutting out these items can result in slimming down an overweight child over time.

Sugar and oral health: High and/or regular consumption of non-milk extrinsic sugar (NMES) foods and drinks is linked with an increased risk of dental caries, gum disease and, in the case of certain drinks, with the erosion of tooth enamel.

Sugar and diabetes: A diet high in sugar can be a factor in promoting insulin resistance – a condition where insulin (a hormone that converts blood sugars into energy and has other roles) is produced by the body in ever-increasing amounts to deal with the sugars in the bloodstream. Eventually its action is weakened or its response is blunted so that, over time, more and more insulin is needed in order to clear the blood of sugars. Eventually this can lead to diabetes.

Sugar and other nutrients: As sugar offers little except calories, a high-sugar diet that is low in more nutritious foods could possibly lead to a child developing malnutrition, with shortfalls in protein, vitamins, minerals, essential fatty acids, for example... while possibly being overweight!

How to cut the sugar in your child's diet

→ Always read the label! Sugar is contained in a great many processed foods – even ready-made salads, such as coleslaw, and breads contain sugars. Get in the habit of reading the labels and, if there is a nutrition panel, see how much sugar there is in a portion. Also check the ingredients list. All the following names are other names for sugar: glucose, dextrose, glucose syrup, lactose, maltose, treacle. And remember the higher up the list they come, the more there is in the product.

→ Avoid giving your child too much fruit juice, as well as the obvious sugary soft drinks. The sugar in juice doesn't count as 'intrinsic' as it does in whole fruit, and it is bad for children's teeth – and high in calories. Offer water or very diluted juice instead.

→ Try to get into the habit of giving children a low-sugar diet right from weaning. Small children need more fat than adults, but they don't need a lot of sugar. Try to give them sweet tastes in natural products, such as fresh and dried fruits.

→ Homemade cakes and bakes are likely to contain a lot less sugar then commercial varieties. Try adding prune or apricot purée to cakes instead of a lot of sugar. Simmer the dried fruits in a little water until tender, cool and purée in a blender, then use in your recipe to replace an equal amount of sugar.

→ If buying any commercial food that has a reduced-sugar version, opt for it – you can save a lot of grams of sugar a day by doing this. But, in general, try to buy fewer of the ready-made, high-sugar products.

→ Trying to ban your child from sweets rarely works. Instead, either give a certain amount of pocket money for sweets and stick to it, or allocate a time (say, straight after supper) when children can have a small amount of sweets. They should then wait half an hour before cleaning their teeth thoroughly.

→ Choose low-sugar varieties of breakfast cereal and add a little sweetness, if necessary, with chopped fresh fruit or a little dried fruit.

→ Reduce the sugar in your child's diet slowly. This is more likely to work in the long run. Children who are used to a low-sugar diet find sweet foods, such as sweets and sugary drinks, too sweet for their taste buds. It usually takes about 2 months to effect the change.

Why do children love sugar?

Young children are thought to enjoy sweet tastes because breast milk is sweet. There are then two main schools of thought about why this liking for sweet things continues. One is that sugar may be difficult to resist because eating sweet food causes the brain's levels of opiates to increase. These stimulate dopamine – a 'happy' chemical, like serotonin.

Other experts believe that a liking for sugar is a learned habit, like a taste for salt, with an added element of 'reward', i.e. sweet foods are often used as treats, bribes, rewards for good behaviour, or instant remedies for a cut or a disappointment. So, they are linked in a child's mind with something desirable or comforting. And, of course, shops are full of sugary foods and drinks, and items with 'hidden' sugar.

See also: Diabetes p151, Obesity p189, Teeth and Gums p209.

Supplements

As a general rule, food supplements in the form of pills, drops and so on shouldn't be necessary for healthy children following a normal balanced diet. If for any reason you are considering supplements for a child with a good diet, it is best to discuss the reasons for doing so with your doctor who will advise you and/or put you in touch with a dietitian.

Supplementing when you don't really know what you're doing is fraught with possible problems and may do more harm than good. What's more, if a supplement really is necessary, in the UK it should be provided for children free, via the NHS.

Dangers of supplements

→ There is a risk of overdosing on some nutrients if the maximum recommended intake is overstepped. Single vitamin A doses of only 100mg can be harmful for children. High intakes of vitamin D can lead to failure to thrive in children. High doses of vitamin B6 can cause nerve problems, and high doses of vitamin C can cause diarrhoea. Excess zinc can hinder absorption of other minerals. And so on. If you are providing your child with any supplement, you must ensure that it is taken at the recommended dosage.

→ Sometimes supplements can interfere with the action of prescription drugs. For example, calcium supplements can interact with some antibiotics; fish oils can react with Warfarin.

→ Herbal supplements, such as echinacea or gingko biloba, should not be given to children.

→ The Food Standards Agency advises against supplements containing chromium picolinate.

Supplements that may be given to children

→ **Vitamin D for small children:** Children under 2 may be given vitamin D supplements (those provided on the NHS also contain vitamins C and A), although most children receive an adequate intake from the diet or the sun. In practice, deficiency is only likely if the child rarely gets outdoors, or is given cows' milk rather than formula milk or breast milk before weaning.

→ **Multi-vitamins/minerals:** May be given to children with eating problems and/or failure to thrive. Such children should be in the care of a physician anyway.

→ **Supplements for vegans or children on special diets:** Given to those who may run the risk of lack of certain nutrients in the diet – for example, iron, calcium and vitamin B12 may be deficient in vegan children.

In addition, children with ADHD, autism, eczema, asthma, behavioural problems or learning difficulties may benefit from omega-3 fish oil supplements. As this is quite a new area of medical research, your doctor may not suggest supplements even if your child has one, or a combination, of these problems. There is no harm in giving your child a 100mg-a-day omega-3 supplement, especially if he or she doesn't eat oily fish. The only contraindication is if a person is on Warfarin or other anti-blood clotting drugs, but this normally applies to older people.

See also: ADHD p134, Anaemia p135, Asthma p137, Autism p138, Behavioural Problems p139, Brain Power p141, Eczema p155, Essential Fatty Acids p156, Minerals p185, Phytochemicals p195, Vitamins p213.

Sweetcorn

Sweetcorn is a favourite of children, partly because it is naturally sweet. It contains good amounts of vitamin C, folate and the carotenoids, zeaxanthin and lutein. Keep cooking times short to retain folate and vitamin C. Cooking with a little oil helps the carotenes to be absorbed – stir-fry baby corn or serve corn on the cob with a little butter.

Teeth and gums

About one in six children under school age has signs of tooth decay and/or erosion.

Dietary factors in tooth decay and erosion

Sugar: When sugary foods or drinks are eaten, the bacteria in the mouth feed on the sugar. This produces acid which, if left in contact with the teeth for long, can cause the tooth enamel to dissolve and, eventually, cavities to form. Starches (e.g. bread and biscuits) can also be broken down by the mouth bacteria. Sugars mixed with starches (e.g. in sweet biscuits) are particularly linked with decay.
Acid: The acids in some foods and drinks, such as fizzy carbonated drinks (high in phosphoric acid), fruit juice and children's yoghurts, can soften the enamel surface of the tooth, causing erosion.

Keeping a child's teeth and gums healthy

→ Brush teeth with fluoride children's paste as soon as teeth appear. Supervise twice-daily brushing at least until 7 years of age. If the teeth aren't properly cleaned, plaque – largely made up of bacteria – can form at the gum margins and will, if not removed regularly, form tartar, a hard deposit which can cause inflammation, bleeding and gum disease. The British Dental Association (BDA) says that children's teeth shouldn't be flossed.
→ Offer water or milk to drink rather than soft drinks and juices. If acidic and/or sugary drinks are offered, give them at meal-times. Small children shouldn't be allowed to sip sweet drinks from drink cups or bottles over long periods nor be given such drinks at bedtime. Acidic drinks bathe a child's mouth in the acids, which can destroy tooth enamel.
→ After acidic or sugary drinks don't brush the teeth for at least 20–30 minutes, because the drink will soften the tooth enamel surface – immediate brushing could cause 'accelerated abrasion' or increased wear on the enamel.
→ Restrict the amount of sugary foods in the diet and, when given, encourage your child to eat them in one go rather than chewing them over a period of time. Whole fruits contain both sugar and acids, but crunching on fresh fruit increases saliva in the mouth, which may cancel out some of the effects of the acids. It is a good idea to get your child to rinse his or her mouth out with water after eating fruit.
→ Sticky foods containing sugar and/or starch, such as toffee and chocolate, cling to teeth and have the potential to cause more damage.
→ Frozen ice lollies should be limited. When frozen, the acids which attack tooth enamel take longer to neutralize in the mouth.
→ Frequent eating of yoghurts and fromage frais can contribute to enamel erosion and tooth decay – the bacteria in the milk react with the lactose (milk sugar) to produce acids.

Other oral problems

Ulcers: Most mouth ulcers have no obvious cause, though there is some evidence that a deficiency in vitamin B12, folate or iron may be a factor.

Bad breath: Good mouth hygiene usually prevents bad breath in children, but other causes could be illness (e.g. throat infection, bronchitis) or constipation. Unexplained bad breath that continues for more than a few days should be investigated by your doctor.

Bleeding gums: Frequent bleeding gums may be a sign of vitamin C deficiency.

Tomatoes

All tomatoes are rich in lycopene, an antioxidant phytochemical that protects against heart disease and cancers and can also help to build strong bones. Canned tomatoes have a similar nutrient profile, though slightly lower in fibre and vitamin C; but on the plus side the lycopene in canned and cooked tomatoes is better absorbed than from fresh raw ones. Tomatoes also contain beta-carotene (which converts to vitamin A in the body), along with vitamin C and E, so they are a source of the powerful 'ACE' group of antioxidant vitamins.

Tips for serving children tomatoes

→ Cherry tomatoes are ideal for young children – either whole in a lunch-box or mixed with cucumber for a side salad.

→ Frying, grilling or roasting tomatoes enhances their sweetness and most children like cooked tomatoes. Fry in good-quality oil to increase the vitamin E value.

→ Add canned or fresh chopped tomatoes to stews, casseroles or soups. Tomato pastes, purées, passata and juice are also all rich sources of antioxidants.

See also: Antioxidants p135, Phytochemicals p195.

Underweight

All children differ, and averages are just that, so if your child falls under the average weight for his height/age but is still within the normal range, that is fine. If he or she is beneath that, a doctor will be able to advise you if there could be a problem.

Being slim or 'skinny' is partly down to inherited genes, so if both parents are naturally thin (or were as children), then it is likely that their offspring will also be slim. Some children are more active, and burn off more energy (calories). If either of these is the case and your child seems strong, with a good bone structure and of reasonable height, slimness should not be a problem. Indeed, on balance it is probably better for a child to be slightly on the lean side than overweight.

Some children, however, have a smaller appetite than others, or an eating problem, and so take in fewer calories and can get thin that way. Growing children need a variety of nutrients in the right amounts to grow, build muscle and bone, and be healthy. If a child is taking in too few calories he or she is likely also to be taking in too few nutrients and thus may not be giving his or her body the chance to develop peak bone mass, as one example (see Bone Health page 141). So for a child who is a poor eater, follow your doctor's advice.

Occasionally, children can fluctuate in their weight. For instance, if they are going through an illness/convalescence lasting several weeks they may lose weight. And weight gain throughout childhood is rarely steady – there are growth spurts and times when a child eats more, and eats less.

Sometimes low weight can be an indication of an underlying condition (e.g. diabetes, Crohn's disease) – which is why it is important to see your doctor about very low weight or failure to thrive. A child who is thin because of an eating problem needs professional help.

Tips for weight gain

If your child needs to gain some weight, and you don't have a specific diet plan from your doctor or dietician, these tips will help:

→ Follow a basic healthy diet plan for your child's age (refer to the Eating Plans on pages 26-31, 58-66 and 119-121), but provide extra calories in the form of extra/larger snacks and calorific drinks. Children who need to gain weight often can't face large meals, so simply increasing portion sizes is rarely the answer – but it's fine to do so if your child can eat more.

→ Ideal snacks are nuts and seeds (for those over 5), dried fruits and handfuls of muesli.

→ A diet very high in fat isn't recommended for any schoolchild, but as fat contains more calories per gram than other nutrients, it is useful to increase the amount of foods that contain higher amounts of the healthy polyunsaturated and monounsaturated fats in order to help a child put on weight. Nuts and seeds (for over 5's) can be added to soups, casseroles, salads and so on, to add calories. Oily fish are also much higher in calories than white fish, and contain more nutrients.

→ Increasing the complex carbohydrate content of a child's diet may also help to put on weight – offer good-quality breads, muesli, oatcakes and tea breads. Potatoes, pasta and rice are all fairly high in calories and can be mixed with, or drizzled with, olive oil or similar to increase the calorie content.

→ Many children like savoury white sauces, like cheese or parsley sauce. These are high in calcium and can be added to white fish, ham, pasta, roast vegetables, for example, to increase the calorie value of a meal.

→ Drinks can provide many calories and nutrients. Milk is ideal as it contains protein and calcium as well as calories – go for whole milk, or homemade milkshakes. At night-time, offer hot milk or hot chocolate or a malted drink about half an hour before bedtime, then get the child to brush his or her teeth just before bed. Fortified milky drinks, containing calories and a range of nutrients and tasting quite pleasant, are available. Juices are also higher in calories than you would think (though they have drawbacks).

→ Try to avoid giving a lot of extra sweets, chocolate and other sugary foods to help weight gain – they contain few nutrients and are not good for the teeth.

→ Don't forget still to offer plenty of fruits and vegetables – though they don't usually contain a lot of calories, they are vital for health.

See also: Appetite Loss p136, Convalescence p149, Illness, feeding during p180, Milk p184, Nuts p188, Obesity p189, Seeds p204, Teeth and Gums p209.

Vegetables

Most vegetables are very low in fat, don't contain a great deal of protein and are low or moderate in calories and starch. Almost all vegetables are a good source of dietary fibre, including soluble fibre. Vegetables contain a wide range of vitamins and minerals. Many are good sources of beta-carotene, vitamin C and folate and potassium, while some – especially leafy green vegetables – are good sources of calcium and iron. More detailed information can be found under specific entries (e.g. Greens –leafy, Potatoes, Root Vegetables). Potatoes are classed as a carbohydrate food and not covered here.

Vegetables are also a major source of phytochemicals – natural plant chemicals that can have potent effects in protecting health. Another bonus is that very few vegetables are common causes of food allergies in children.

Five-a-day

Two to three portions of vegetables should go towards making up your child's daily 'five-a-day' intake of fruit and vegetables – and yet few children meet this target.

Fresh, frozen or canned vegetables can count, as can cooked vegetables, as long as they make up a portion. Many manufactured foods, including vegetable soups and ready meals will contain vegetables that can count – sometimes this information is included on the label. However, it is best to for your child to derive as many 'five-a-day' vegetables as possible from home-cooked meals – ideally prepared with fresh vegetables.

Try to vary your child's intake as much as possible; aim for at least one salad portion a day and for as wide a variety of different colours as possible. Although pulses are not strictly vegetables, one portion a day can count towards a child's five-a-day unless that portion is providing the protein in your meal, then it won't count as a fruit or veg portion too. Baked beans in tomato sauce and canned pulses can count as a veg portion with the same proviso, but try to choose low-sugar, low-salt varieties of baked beans, and pulses canned without added salt if possible.

Tips on serving children vegetables

→ There is little appeal or nutritional merit in overcooked vegetables – serve them steamed, lightly boiled, baked, microwaved, sautéed or as part of a stir-fry to retain colour, texture, visual appeal and maximum vitamins.

→ Children often find vegetable mixes more appetising than one large serving of a single vegetable, so mix and match when you can. Try purées of two vegetables (carrot and parsnip for example) or stir-fries (e.g. beans, carrot, sweetcorn and shredded cabbage).

→ For children who don't like their leafy greens, purée them into soups, shred them into casseroles and add them to stir-fries.

→ Chunks of vegetable cooked in the roasting pan under a meat joint are delicious – the meat juices drip down on to them and the fats from the meat will help the carotenes in the vegetables to be absorbed.

→ For reluctant veg eaters, vegetable soups are ideal, as they can be puréed and/or mixed with other flavours – e.g. cheese, chicken.

→ Aim for one salad a day. If your child dislikes leafy salad, grate vegetables such as carrots, beetroot or firm cabbage together and toss in a dressing, or cut vegetables into batons and serve with a dip. Don't slice, chop or grate vegetables until just before they are needed as the cut edges will oxidize and they will lose vitamin C.

→ Adding vegetables to meat dishes broadens the nutritional profile and reduces its total fat content (because you use less meat).

Using vegetables to extend meat and other dishes:

→ Finely chopped tomatoes, carrots, onion, celery or mushrooms are ideal to add to minced meat dishes, such as cottage pie, pasta sauce and chilli con carne.

→ Chopped or shredded cabbage, swede, parsnips, peppers, broad beans and broccoli florets are ideal to add bulk and flavour to stews and casseroles.

→ Small chunks of cauliflower, squash or aubergine, or whole spinach leaves, work well in curries and other spiced dishes.

→ Add broccoli and sweetcorn to chicken stir-fries, mushrooms and Chinese leaves (e.g. pak choi) to beef stir-fries, mixed peppers to pork stir-fries.

→ Mix suitable vegetables into rice dishes – for example petit pois or sweetcorn kernels.

→ Fill halved and scooped-out beef tomatoes with a meat or vegetarian mix and bake with a cheese and breadcrumb topping.

See also: Carbohydrates p144, Dietary Fibre p152, Food Allergies p162, Fruit p173, Minerals p185, Phytochemicals p195, Vitamins p213.

Vitamins

Vitamins are organic compounds present in minute quantities in the diet, which are essential for bodily health and day-to-day functioning.

Vitamins B group and C are water-soluble, meaning that excess intake is excreted in the urine and also that they are leached out of foods when water is used in their preparation or cooking. These vitamins need to be taken on a regular basis as they cannot be stored in the body. Vitamins A, D, E and K are fat-soluble, meaning that they can be stored in the body and surplus is not excreted in the urine.

Each of the eleven vitamins has a different role to play in the body and deficiencies can cause all kinds of growth and health problems. To ensure that a child's diet contains recommended amounts of all the vitamins, a varied, balanced diet is required. If this is in place, there is little need for a parent to pore over vitamin charts, although it is useful to have a working knowledge of which foods are good sources of which vitamins. If a child eats only a small range of foods – as some do, especially when young – you can see which vitamins they may be lacking and discover alternative sources.

Vitamins, like minerals, are best absorbed in foods rather than as supplements. The charts on the following pages give the role of the various vitamins and lists those foods that are good sources.

See also: Antioxidants p135, Phytochemicals p195, Supplements p208.

VITAMINS

Vitamin	What it does	Deficiency can cause
Vitamin A (retinol) and retinol equivalents (alpha- and beta-carotene)	Vision, healthy eyes, skin and growth.	Poor night vision and eye problems and poor resistance to infection.
Vitamin B1 (thiamin)	Helps to release carbohydrate from foods and ensures supply of glucose to the brain and nerves.	The disease beri beri.
Vitamin B2 (riboflavin)	Helps release fat and protein from the food that we eat and convert it for use as energy and lean tissue. Maintains healthy skin and mucous membrane.	Eye and mouth problems.
Vitamin B3 (niacin)	Helps to release energy from food and requirement is related to the amount of energy expended.	Pellagra, a sunburn-like skin complaint which is rare but can be fatal.
Vitamin B6 (pyridoxine)	Important player in the metabolization of protein and helps the body to manufacture vitamin B3 (niacin) from the amino acid tryptophan if necessary; helps blood health.	Along with deficiencies in B12 and folate, a B6 deficiency plays a part in causing high levels of the amino acid homocysteine in the blood, which is linked with heart disease.
Vitamin B12	Necessary for the formation of blood cells and nerves.	Pernicious anaemia, nerve damage, and with B6 and folate deficiencies it can contribute to high blood homocysteine levels (see B6).
Folate	Vital for formation of blood cells and infant development.	Birth defects, such as spina bifida; megaloblastic anaemia, and with B6 and B12 deficiency can contribute to high blood homocysteine levels (see B6).

Found in	Notes	Recommended daily amounts
Retinol is found in liver, dairy produce, eggs and oily fish. Carotenes can be converted to vitamin A in the body, and they are found in red, orange, yellow and dark green fruits and vegetables. In addition, the carotenes are an important group of phytochemicals with antioxidant powers.	Excess vitamin A is toxic. It can be stored in the liver and can cause liver and bone damage, and other problems. Excess is linked with birth defects and so should be avoided in pregnancy (no more than 3,300mcg/day). Daily intake should not exceed 900mcg in infants; 1800mcg aged 1–3; and 3000mcg aged 4–6. Beta-carotene is not toxic as excess is excreted, although more than 30mg a day may colour the skin orange.	0–12 months 350mcg 1–3 years 400mcg 4–6 years 500mcg
A variety of foods, including pork, bacon, fortified breakfast cereals and nuts.	Excess not harmful. As B vitamins are water-soluble they can be leached from food during prolonged simmering.	0–9 months 0.2mg 10–12 months 0.3mg 1–3 years 0.5mg 4–6 years 0.7mg
Offal, fortified breakfast cereals, dairy produce.	Water-soluble vitamin; no upper safe limits.	0–12 months 0.4mg 1–3 years 0.6mg 4–6 years 0.8mg
Yeast extract, liver, meat, fish and fortified breakfast cereals.	Very high intakes can cause liver and kidney damage, which is reversible if B3 intake is withdrawn.	0–6 months 3mg 7–9 months 4mg 10–12 months 5mg 1–3 years 8mg 4–6 years 11mg
Meat, fish, eggs, whole grains, fortified cereals, some vegetables.	Very high doses are inadvisable as they can cause nerve damage.	0–6 months 0.2mg 7–9 months 0.3mg 10–12 months 0.4mg 1–3 years 0.7mg 4–6 years 0.9mg
Meat, fish, animal produce, seaweed.	Vegans may need a supplement as B12 is only found in animal produce, apart from seaweed.	0–6 months 0.3mcg 6–12 months 0.4mcg 1–3 years 0.5mcg 4–6 years 0.8mcg
Offal, leafy greens, whole grains, nuts, pulses, fortified breakfast cereals.	Very high folate intake may hinder absorption of zinc. New research indicates that folate supplements in pregnancy can lower the chances of a child developing leukaemia.	0–12 months 50mcg 1–3 years 70mcg 4–6 years 100mcg

VITAMINS - CONTINUED

Vitamin	What it does	Deficiency can cause
Vitamin C	Antioxidant vitamin helps boost immune system; builds healthy connective tissue, bones and teeth, helps wound and fracture healing, helps iron absorption.	Bleeding gums, poor wound healing, low resistance to infection and, eventually, scurvy, which is now very rare in Western society.
Vitamin D (cholecalciferol)	Helps mineral absorption in the body and therefore vital for building bone.	Rickets in children.
Vitamin E (tocopherol)	Antioxidant vitamin which protects cell membranes and helps prevent plaque build up in the arteries; thins the blood and thus helps prevent heart disease; boosts the immune system and may protect against cancers; helps boost skin condition, healing and fertility. Also prevents polyunsaturated fats from oxidizing.	Blood problems in premature infants, nerve problems in older children.
Vitamin K	Essential for normal blood clotting.	Rare but may occur in cystic fibrosis or liver disease. Deficiency at birth can cause bleeding disorders.

Found in	Notes	Recommended daily amounts
Fruits and vegetables, especially blackcurrants, citrus fruits, strawberries, guava, papaya, kiwi fruit, sweet peppers and leafy green vegetables.	Extra vitamin C may be needed when the body is under stress. This water-soluble vitamin needs to be taken regularly as the body cannot store it. High doses of vitamin C can produce a laxative effect and/or stomach irritation. Vitamin C is best taken in the form of real food rather than supplements. Many experts feel that the RDAs for vitamin C may be too low – certainly moderately higher intakes may be beneficial and 60–100mg a day may be a better target for schoolchildren.	0–12 months 25mg 1–6 years 30mg
Eggs, oily fish, fortified breakfast cereals, fortified margarines. Vitamin D is also manufactured in the body by the action of sunlight on the skin.	This fat-soluble vitamin is necessary in the diet in the early years of a child's life; later, sunlight normally provides enough for children. Excess vitamin D causes kidney damage and other problems.	0–6 months 8.5mcg 7–12 months 7mcg 1–3 years 7mcg 4 and over – no dietary need
Leafy green vegetables, whole grains, nuts, seeds, butter, egg yolk, poultry, seafood.	Requirement for vitamin E is closely linked with intake of polyunsaturated oils – the higher the fat intake, the more vitamin E is required. Because of this the UK doesn't set RDAs for vitamin E.	
Widespread, but green leafy vegetables are a major source.	Vitamin K can be synthesized in the body so no RDAs have been set. However, some new born babies are deficient and therefore supplements are routinely given at birth.	

Water

Infants who are being breast-fed or who are on formula milk don't need much in the way of extra fluids, but once they start on solids they will need to increase their fluid intake. Water is the ideal fluid to add to their milk allowance as it doesn't contribute to tooth decay or over-consumption of calories.

Schoolchildren should drink about 6–8 glasses of fluid a day, more if it's hot or if they are exercising a lot. Regular water intake can help to prevent constipation and if you can get children used to drinking water at an early age rather than sugary and/or acidic soft drinks (including juice) this may be of long-term benefit both to their weight and dental health.

See also: Drinks for Infants p24, Constipation p148, Drinks p153, Milk p184, Teeth and Gums p209.

WHEAT
see Grains

Whole foods

'Whole foods' is a term used to describe food which is in its natural, unadulterated form – e.g. whole grains, fresh fruits and vegetables, nuts, seeds and pulses. As a general rule, whole unprocessed or minimally processed foods should form a significant part of the older child's diet as they are likely to contain more vitamins, minerals and dietary fibre, and fewer of the not-so-good things, such as saturated fat, sugar and additives. They also take more chewing and can be more satisfying. Children raised on a whole-food diet may have less of a taste for sweets and snacks.

See also: Health Foods p178, Processed Foods p199.

Yoghurt and fromage frais

Yoghurt and fromage frais can be good sources of calcium for children, but full-fat varieties contain over half of their calories as fat, a significant amount of which is saturated. Many yoghurts aimed at children contain a good deal of added sugar or fruit sugars, and the speciality varieties containing items such as crunchy sweets, chocolate chips, etc., are not the healthy foods some parents perceive them to be. They may also contain several food additives and 'fruit flavours' are just that – flavourings not real fruit.

Go for natural yoghurt or fromage frais and add puréed fruits yourself, or drizzle honey over the top. Younger children can enjoy full-fat yoghurt, but as children's fat needs decline it is best to choose the lower-fat varieties. Bio yoghurts contain natural bacteria which help to keep the gut colonized and thus aid digestion, and can help to prevent both constipation and diarrhoea. If children are having to take antibiotics, these will kill off the good bacteria in the gut, and bio yoghurt can help to replace them.

Yoghurt may be tolerated even by children who are intolerant of cows' milk as the fermentation process aids digestion. Greek yoghurt made from ewes' milk is also useful. Soya 'yoghurt' is an alternative for vegans but unless specifically labelled as 'calcium-fortified', it will contain only around a tenth of the calcium a low-fat natural yoghurt, for example, will provide.

See also: Dairy Produce p150, Food Additives p159, Teeth and Gums p209.

CONTACTS

ALLERGY UK
No 3, White Oak Square, London
Road, Swanley, Kent BR8 7AG
Tel: helpline 01322 619864
Web: www.allergyuk.org
Email: info@allergyuk.org

THE ANAPHYLAXIS CAMPAIGN
PO Box 275, Farnborough,
Hampshire GU14 6SX
Tel: helpline 01252 542029
Web: www.anaphylaxis.org.uk

ASTHMA UK
Summit House, 70 Wilson Street,
London EC2A 2DB
Tel: helpline 08457 010203;
other 020 7786 4900
Web: www.asthma.org.uk
Email: info@asthma.org.uk

**THE BRITISH DIETETIC
ASSOCIATION**
5th Floor, Charles House,
148–9 Great Charles Street,
Queensway, Birmingham B3 3HT
Tel: 0121 200 8080
Web: www.bda.uk.com
Email: info@bda.uk.com

CancerBACUP
3 Bath Place, Rivington Street,
London EC2A 3JR
Tel: helpline 0808 800 1234
Web: www.cancerbacup.org.uk

INSTITUTE OF CHILD HEALTH
30 Guildford Street, London WC1N 1EH
Tel: 020 7242 9789
Web: www.ich.ucl.ac.uk
Email: info@gosh.nhs.uk

COELIAC UK
PO Box 220, High Wycombe,
Bucks HP11 2HY
Tel: helpline 0870 444 8804;
office 01494 437278
Web: www.coeliac.co.uk
Email: diet@coeliac.co.uk

DIABETES UK
10 Parkway, London NW1 7AA
Tel: 020 7424 1000
Web: www.diabetes.org.uk
Email: info@diabetes.org.uk

**THE BRITISH DYSLEXIA
ASSOCIATION**
98 London Road, Reading RG1 5AU
Tel: helpline 0118 966 8271
office 0118 966 2677
Email: helpline@bdadyslexia.org.uk
Web: www.bda-dyslexia.org.uk

THE DYSPRAXIA FOUNDATION
8 West Alley, Hitchin, Herts SG5 1EG
Tel: helpline 01462 454 986;
general enquiries 01462 455 016
Web: www.dyspraxiafoundation.org.uk

NATIONAL ECZEMA SOCIETY
Hill House, Highgate Hill,
London N19 5NA
Tel: helpline 0870 241 3604;
office 020 7281 3553
Web: www.eczema.org
Email: helpline@eczema.org

THE FOOD COMMISSION
94 White Lion Street, London N1 9PF
Tel: 020 7837 2250
Web: www.foodcomm.org.uk
Email: enquiries@foodcomm.org.uk

THE DEPARTMENT OF HEALTH
Richmond House, 79 Whitehall,
London SW1A 2NL
Tel: 020 7210 4850
Web: www.doh.gov.uk
Email: dhmail@dh.gsi.gov.uk

BRITISH HEART FOUNDATION
14 Fitzhardinge Street,
London W1H 6DH
Tel: infoline 08450 708070;
office 020 7935 0185
Web: www.bhf.org.uk
Email: internet@bhf.org.uk

**THE HYPERACTIVE CHILDREN'S
SUPPORT GROUP**
71 Whyke Lane, Chichester,
West Sussex PO19 7PD
Tel: 01243 539966
Web: www.hacsg.org.uk
Email: hyperactive@hacsg.org.uk

**BRITISH NUTRITION
FOUNDATION**
High Holborn House,
52–54 High Holborn,
London WC1V 6RQ
Tel: 020 7404 6504
Web: www.nutrition.org.uk
Email: postbox@nutrition.org.uk

**THE ASSOCIATION FOR THE
STUDY OF OBESITY**
20 Brook Meadow Close,
Woodford Green, Essex IG8 9NR
Tel: 07767 365718
Web: www.aso.org.uk
Email: oric@aso.org.uk

**THE SOIL ASSOCIATION
(organic food)**
Bristol House, 40–56 Victoria Street,
Bristol, BS1 6BY
Tel: 0117 314 5000
Web: www.soilassociation.org
Email: info@soilassociation.org

THE VEGETARIAN SOCIETY
Parkdale, Dunham Road,
Altrincham, Cheshire WA14 4QG
Tel: 0161 925 2000
Web: www.vegsoc.org
Email: info@vegsoc.org

FOOD STANDARDS AGENCY UK
Aviation House, 125 Kingsway,
London WC2B 6NH
Tel: 020 7276 8000
Email:
helpline@foodstandards.gsi.gov.uk
Web: www.food.gov.uk

Index

additives *see* food additives
ADHD (attention deficit
    hyperactivity disorder), 134
allergies, 162–4
    asthma, 137–8
    cows'-milk protein, 184
    eczema, 155
    hay fever, 177–8
    in infants, 10, 22–3
    nuts, 162, 163–4, 189
    peanuts, 22, 23, 56, 162, 189,
        195
    toddlers and pre-school
        children, 56
almonds: fruit and nut pasta salad,
    122
amino acids, 108, 199–200
anaemia, 135
anaphylactic shock, 163
antibiotics, 171, 180, 185, 194
antioxidants, 135
anxiety, 135–6
appetite loss, 136–7
appetite size, 56
apples, 137
    apple muffins, 99
    apple smoothie, 102
    fruit and nut pasta salad, 122
apricots: apricot and brown rice
    salad, 123
    fruit and nut cookies, 131
asthma, 137–8
autism, 138

babies *see* infants
bacteria: food poisoning, 166–7
    in milk, 185
    oral health, 209
    probiotics, 180
bad breath, 210
baked beans, homemade, 75
bananas, 138
    banana bread, 101
    banana split, 97
    berry and banana milkshake,
        103
    fresh fruit trifles, 96
barbecues, 169, 177
batch cooking, 14, 115

beans, 200–1
    canned pulses, 144
    chunky vegetable and bean
        soup, 69
    homemade baked beans in
        tomato sauce, 75
    vegetable and butter bean
        hotpot, 76
bedwetting, 138–9
beef: basic minced beef, 89
    beef and carrot casserole, 88
    beef and vegetable hash, 43
    beef stock, 89
    cottage pie, 89
    homemade burgers, 86
behavioural problems, 139–40
berry and banana milkshake, 103
berry fruits, 140
biscuits: fruit and nut cookies, 131
bleeding gums, 210
blood sugar levels, 110, 139, 142
Body Mass Index (BMI), 190
bones, 141
bottle-feeding, 10–12, 22, 24
brain power, 141–2
bread, 142–3
breakfast: school children, 110–11
    see also eating plans
breast-feeding, 10–12, 22, 24
broccoli: creamed pasta with
    vegetables, 36
    macaroni and broccoli cheese,
        35
    potato and vegetable gratin, 34
burgers: homemade burgers, 86
    vegetable burgers, 126
butter beans: vegetable and butter
    bean hotpot, 76
buying food, 167

caffeine, 142
cakes, 112
    banana bread, 101
    carrot cake, 100
    date loaf, 98
calcium, 185, 186–7
    and bone health, 141
    dairy produce, 145, 150
    toddlers and pre-school
        children, 54
    vegan diet, 13, 108

vegetarian diet, 13, 108
calories: fats, 157
    food labelling, 165
    and overweight, 189
    toddlers and pre-school
        children, 50
campylobacter, 166
cancer prevention, 143
canned foods, 143–4
carbohydrates, 144–5
    food pyramid, 52–3
    Glycaemic Index, 191–2
    packed lunches, 112
    sugars, 205–7
    toddlers and pre-school
        children, 53, 54
carbonated drinks, 153–4
carrots, 145
    beef and carrot casserole, 88
    carrot and orange soup, 68
    carrot cake, 100
casseroles: beef and carrot
    casserole, 88
    chicken casserole, 41
    vegetable and butter bean
        hotpot, 76
cereals, 13, 175
cheese, 53, 145–6, 150
    cheese dip, 72
    cheese sauce, 46
    cod, potato and Cheddar pie, 40
    creamed pasta with vegetables,
        36
    fish and tomato bake, 39
    Greek cheese and spinach pie,
        94
    macaroni and broccoli cheese,
        35
    potato and vegetable gratin, 34
    traditional pizza, 79
    tuna, pasta and tomato bake,
        80
chicken: chicken and mushroom
    pasta, 42
    chicken and pasta salad, 124
    chicken and vegetable pie, 85
    chicken casserole, 41
    chicken dippers, 84
    chicken enchiladas, 128
    chicken soup, 70
    chicken stock, 41

chickpeas: hummus, 73
    vegetable burgers, 126
chips, 81, 198
choking, on nuts, 189
cholesterol, 146, 158
chromium, 185, 188
citrus fruits, 147
Clostridium perfringens, 166
cobalt, 185
cod, 159
    cod, potato and Cheddar pie, 40
    fish and tomato bake, 39
    fish fingers with potato wedges,
        81
coeliac disease, 22, 147
colds, 147–8
colic, 148
constipation, 148–9
convalescence, 149–50
convenience foods, 115–17
cookies, fruit and nut, 131
cooking: encouraging children, 114
    food safety, 168
    fried food, 172
    grilled food, 172, 177
    microwaves, 183
copper, 185
cottage pie, 89
coughs, 147–8
cows'-milk protein allergy, 184
crisps, homemade vegetable, 71
crumble, plum, 130
custard: canned, 144
    fresh fruit trifles, 96

dairy produce, 53, 150
    after weaning, 13
    alternatives, 150
    packed lunches, 112
date loaf, 98
dehydration, 140, 142, 151
delinquency, 140
diabetes, 151–2, 206
dietary fibre, 106, 149, 152
digestive problems: coeliac
        disease, 22, 147
    colic, 148
    constipation, 148–9
    stomach upsets, 205
dips: cheese dip, 72
    chicken dippers, 84

hummus, 73
dried fruits, 153
drinks, 153–4
    apple smoothie, 102
    berry and banana milkshake,
        103
    dehydration, 140, 142, 151
    for infants, 24
    labels, 164
    packed lunches, 112
    toddlers and pre-school
        children, 51
    yoghurt smoothie, 103
    see also water
dyslexia and dyspraxia, 154

E coli, 166
E numbers, 160–1, 166
eating out, food safety, 168–9
eating plans: infants, 26–31
    school children, 119–21
    toddlers and pre-school
        children, 58–66
eczema, 155
eggs, 156
    baked eggs and peppers, 125
    and MMR vaccine, 163
    salmon and egg flan, 83
    Spanish omelette, 93
    tuna and egg kedgeree, 127
enchiladas, chicken, 128
essential fatty acids, 156–7
evening meals: school children,
        113
    see also eating plans
exercise, 118, 140, 190

fast food, 115–17
fatigue, 182
fats and oils, 157–8
    and cholesterol levels, 146
    dairy produce, 150
    food labelling, 165
    food pyramid, 52–3
    low-fat foods, 193
    in milk, 184
    organic foods, 194
    school children, 106
    toddlers and pre-school
        children, 50
    weaning, 12

fever, 158
fibre, 106, 149, 152
fish, 159
    and brain power, 142
    cod, potato and Cheddar pie, 40
    fish and tomato bake, 39
    fish fingers with potato wedges,
        81
    food safety, 106, 171
    salmon and egg flan, 83
    tuna and potato fishcakes, 38
flan, salmon and egg, 83
flavourings, 160
fluoride, 185, 188, 209
folate, 214–15
food additives, 139, 142, 159–61, 166
food allergies see allergies
food intolerance, 22–3, 162–3
food labelling, 164–6
food poisoning, 166–7
food pyramid, 52–3
food safety see safety
food standards, 170–2
fool, fruit, 97
free radicals, 135
fried food, 172
fromage frais, 218
frozen food, 173
fruit, 173–4
    after weaning, 13
    berry fruits, 140
    canned fruit, 144
    dried fruits, 153
    fruit and nut pasta salad, 122
    fruit fool, 97
    juice, 24, 153, 164
    organic foods, 193–4
    packed lunches, 112
    phytochemicals, 173, 195–7
    purées, 12, 14
    residues in, 170, 194
    summer fruit compote, 96
    toddlers and pre-school
        children, 51, 53, 54
    see also apples; raspberries etc.
fruit and nut cookies, 131
fussy eating, 11, 55–6, 174–5

game, 198–9
genetically modified (GM) foods,
        171–2, 194

gluten intolerance, 22, 23, 143, 147
Glycaemic Index (GI), 191-2
goats' cheese: cheese dip, 72
grains, 175
grapes, 176
Greek cheese and spinach pie, 94
greens, leafy, 176-7
grilled food, 172, 177
gums, bleeding, 210

ham and rice salad, 90
haricot beans: homemade baked beans in tomato sauce, 75
hay fever, 177-8
health foods, 178
heart health, 178
heavy metals, food safety, 171
honey, 179
hotpot, vegetable and butter bean, 76
hummus, 73
hunger, 179-80, 191
hyperactivity, 134

illness: convalescence, 149-50
feeding during, 180
fever, 158
food refusal, 55
immune system, 147-8
infants, 10-47
allergies, 10, 22-3
drinks, 24
eating plans, 26-31
feeding, 13-14
recipes, 32-47
suitable foods, 16-20
weaning, 10-12, 22
insomnia, 180-1
iodine, 185, 186-7
iron, 185, 186-7
anaemia, 135
for infants, 11, 13
toddlers and pre-school children, 51
vegan diet, 108
vegetarian diet, 13, 108

juices, 24, 153, 164
junk food, 56, 116-17

kebabs, lamb and cherry tomato, 129
kedgeree, tuna and egg, 127
kiwi fruit: apple smoothie, 102

labels see food labelling
lactose intolerance, 162, 185
lamb and cherry tomato kebabs, 129
learning problems, 154
lentils: apricot and brown rice salad, 123
lentil ragu, 92
red lentil and tomato soup, 32
lethargy, 182
listeria, 166
lunch: school children, 111-13
see also eating plans

macaroni and broccoli cheese, 35
magnesium, 141, 185, 186-7
manganese, 185
meals, family, 140
see also eating plans
meat, 182-3
after weaning, 13
food labelling, 164
food safety, 167, 168, 169
food standards, 170-1
grilled food, 177
organic foods, 194
poultry and game, 198-9
serving sizes, 53
melon: ham and rice salad, 90
mental abilities, 141-2
autism, 138
breakfast and, 110
dyslexia and dyspraxia, 154
learning problems, 154
microwaves, 183
milk, 153, 184-5
after weaning, 13, 24
berry and banana milkshake, 103
bottle-feeding, 10-12, 22, 24
breast-feeding, 10-12, 24
toddlers and pre-school children, 50, 53, 54
minerals, 185-8
organic foods, 193-4
supplements, 208

MMR vaccine, 163
monounsaturated fats, 157
mouth ulcers, 210
muffins, apple, 99
multi-vitamins, 208
muscle development, 188
mushrooms: chicken and mushroom pasta, 42
lentil ragu, 92

nutrients, 188
nuts, 106, 188-9
nut allergy, 162, 163-4, 189

obesity and overweight, 189-93
and hunger, 179, 191
school children, 117-18
toddlers and pre-school children, 57
weaning and, 10
offal, 183
omega-3 fatty acids, 13, 106, 156-7, 158
omega-6 fatty acids, 156-7, 158
omelette, Spanish, 93
onions, 193
traditional pizza, 79
oranges, 147
carrot and orange soup, 68
organic foods, 115, 193-4
overweight see obesity and overweight

packed lunches, 111-13
pasta: chicken and mushroom pasta, 42
chicken and pasta salad, 124
creamed pasta with vegetables, 36
fruit and nut pasta salad, 122
macaroni and broccoli cheese, 35
pasta shells with peppers, 78
tuna, pasta and tomato bake, 80
peaches: fruit fool, 97
peanut butter: fruit and nut cookies, 131
peanuts, 195
allergy, 22, 23, 56, 162, 189, 195
pears: yoghurt smoothie, 103

peas: creamed pasta with
    vegetables, 36
peppers, 195
    baked eggs and peppers, 125
    chicken and pasta salad, 124
    pasta shells with peppers, 78
pesticide residues, 170–1, 185,
    194
phosphates, 141
phosphorous, 185
phytochemicals, 173, 176–7,
    195–7, 212
picnics, food safety, 169
pies: chicken and vegetable pie, 85
    cod, potato and Cheddar pie, 40
    cottage pie, 89
    Greek cheese and spinach pie,
    94
pineapple: apple smoothie, 102
pizza, traditional, 79
planning meals see eating plans
plum crumble, 130
polyunsaturated fats, 158
portion sizes, 53, 54, 119
potassium, 185, 186–7
potatoes, 198
    beef and vegetable hash, 43
    chips, 81, 198
    cod, potato and Cheddar pie, 40
    cottage pie, 89
    potato and vegetable gratin, 34
    potato cakes, 74
    Spanish omelette, 93
    tuna and potato fishcakes, 38
poultry, 198–9
pre-school children see toddlers
    and pre-school children
probiotics, 180
processed foods, 199
protein, 199–200
    food pyramid, 52–3
    meat, 182–3
    packed lunches, 112
    toddlers and pre-school
    children, 54
    vegan diet, 108
pulses, 144, 200–1
    see also beans
purées, 12, 14

Quorn, 201

ragu, lentil, 92
raspberries: fresh fruit trifles, 96
    fruit fool, 97
    yoghurt smoothie, 103
ready meals, 202
red kidney beans: chunky
    vegetable and bean soup, 69
reheating food, 168
residues, food safety, 170–1, 185,
    194
rice: apricot and brown rice salad,
    123
    canned rice pudding, 144
    ham and rice salad, 90
    tuna and egg kedgeree, 127
root vegetables, 202–3

safety, 167–9
    feeding infants, 14
    fish, 159
    food poisoning, 166–7
    microwaves, 183
    milk, 185
salads: apricot and brown rice
    salad, 123
    chicken and pasta salad, 124
    fruit and nut pasta salad, 122
    ham and rice salad, 90
    packed lunches, 112
salmon, 159
    salmon and egg flan, 83
salmonella, 166
salt, 203–4
    food labelling, 165
    school children, 106
    toddlers and pre-school
    children, 50, 51
saturated fats, 146, 150, 157
sauces: cheese sauce, 46
    tomato sauce, 47
    vegetable sauce, 44
school children, 104–31
    breakfast, 110–11
    eating plans, 119–21
    encouraging healthy eating,
    114–17
    lunch, 111–13
    nutritional needs, 106–8
    recipes, 122–31
    weight control, 117–18
school meals, 111–12

seeds, 204–5
selenium, 185, 186–7
serving sizes, 53, 54, 119
shock, anaphylactic, 163
skin, eczema, 155
sleep problems, 180–1
smoothies: apple smoothie, 102
    yoghurt smoothie, 103
snacks: school children, 11
    toddlers and pre-school
    children, 50, 54, 56
sodium, 185, 203–4
    see also salt
solid foods, introducing, 12, 22
soups: canned soups, 144
    carrot and orange soup, 68
    chicken soup, 70
    chunky vegetable and bean
    soup, 69
    red lentil and tomato soup,
    32
soya, 150, 163–4, 171–2, 201
Spanish omelette, 93
spinach: Greek cheese and
    spinach pie, 94
starches see carbohydrates
stock: beef, 89
    chicken, 41
    vegetable, unsalted, 32
stomach upsets, 205
storing food, 167, 168
strawberries: banana split, 97
    berry and banana milkshake,
    103
    summer fruit compote, 96
stress, 55, 135–6
sugar, 144, 205–7
    and behavioural problems,
    139–40
    food labelling, 166
    and oral health, 206, 209
    sweets, 117
    toddlers and pre-school
    children, 50, 57
sulphur, 185
summer fruit compote, 96
supplements, 208
sweet potatoes: potato and
    vegetable gratin, 34
sweet tooth, 57
sweetcorn, 209

sweeteners, 205-7
sweets, 117

teabreads: banana bread, 101
  date loaf, 98
teeth and gums, 206, 209-10
teething, 55
tiredness, 55, 182
toddlers and pre-school children,
  48-103
  eating plans, 58-66
  feeding problems, 55-7
  feeding strategies, 54
  nutrition, 50-3
  recipes, 68-103
  weight control, 57
tomatoes, 210
  basic minced beef, 89
  beef and carrot casserole, 88
  canned tomatoes, 144
  chicken and pasta salad, 124
  chunky vegetable and bean
    soup, 69
  fish and tomato bake, 39
  homemade baked beans in
    tomato sauce, 75
  lamb and cherry tomato kebabs,
    129
  red lentil and tomato soup, 32
  tomato sauce, 47
  traditional pizza, 79
  tuna, pasta and tomato bake,
    80
tortillas: chicken enchiladas, 128
'traffic light' system, 192
trans fats, 146, 158, 166
trifles, fresh fruit, 96
tuna, 159
  tuna and egg kedgeree, 127
  tuna and potato fishcakes, 38
  tuna, pasta and tomato bake,
    80

ulcers, mouth, 210
underweight children, 210-11

vaccine, MMR, 163
vegan diet: dairy alternatives, 150
  infants, 13
  school children, 108
  supplements, 208

vegetables, 212-13
  after weaning, 13
  beef and vegetable hash, 43
  canned vegetables, 144
  chicken and vegetable pie, 85
  chicken casserole, 41
  chicken soup, 70
  chunky vegetable and bean
    soup, 69
  dislike of, 56
  homemade vegetable crisps,
    71
  leafy greens, 176-7
  organic foods, 193-4
  phytochemicals, 176-7, 195-7,
    212
  purées, 12, 14
  residues in, 170, 194
  root vegetables, 202-3
  toddlers and pre-school
    children, 51, 53, 54
  vegetable and butter bean
    hotpot, 76
  vegetable burgers, 126
  vegetable sauce, 44
  vegetable stock, unsalted, 32
  see also potatoes; tomatoes etc.
vegetarian diet: food labelling,
    164
  infants, 13
  school children, 108
  toddlers and pre-school
    children, 54
vitamins, 213-15
  antioxidants, 135
  organic foods, 193-4
  supplements, 208
vitamin A, 107, 213, 214-15
vitamin B group, 108, 213,
    214-17
vitamin C, 213, 216-17
vitamin D, 11, 141, 208, 213,
    216-17
vitamin E, 213, 216-17
vitamin K, 213, 216-17

water, drinking, 24, 140, 142, 151,
    218
weaning, 10-12, 22
weight: infants, 14
  school children, 117-18

toddlers and pre-school
    children, 57
  underweight children, 210-11
  see also obesity and overweight
whole foods, 218

yoghurt, 53, 218
  banana split, 97
  cheese dip, 72
  fruit fool, 97
  yoghurt smoothie, 103

zinc, 107, 185, 186-7

Acknowledgement

The author and publisher
would like to thank the following
company for assistance with this
publication:
Tumbletots (UK) Limited,
Blue Bird Park, Bromsgrove
Road, Hunnington, Halesowen,
West Midlands C62 0TT:
Tel 0121 585 7003;
www.tumbletots.com